W9-DAJ-584

t'ai-chi chi kung

Coming from a background of twelve years as a general practitioner, I felt aware that there was something lacking in what I was able to offer. I first met Choy over three years ago and attended his workshops. What he had to say seemed immediately to make sense. Since then I have explored many different avenues and teachers, but nowhere has everything made such sense as in Choy's teaching. This book is an excellent introduction to Choy's work. It's so much more than T'ai-Chi, as it shows us how we can start to change our whole way of being, without turning our backs on our ordinary Western lives.

Dr Lynette J Bowden MBBS, DRCOG, MFHom

Peter Chin Kean Choy studied T'ai-Chi Chi Kung with Master Huang of Malaysia. Master Huang was a pupil of Professor Cheng Man-Ching. Choy also learned the application of T'ai-Chi Chi Kung with his father, Chin Ket Leong, who was a Chinese herbal doctor and martial arts Master. He learned the Taoist Sciences with Mantak Chia in Thailand and the Option Process at the Option Institute, Massachusetts, USA. He combined his experience of T'ai-Chi Chi Kung with other Taoist exercises to develop the Rainbow T'ai-Chi Chi Kung Practice and Philosophy. He has led weekly classes and workshops on T'ai-Chi, Chi Kung and the Taoist Arts for the last twenty years. He was a member of the Findhorn Foundations where he started the Rainbow Bridge Journal. He has written many booklets on Foundation T'ai-Chi Chi Kung course subjects.

When I first took up T'ai-Chi Chi Kung , I was coming to the end of an active sports career. Within weeks of beginning with Choy, many of my nagging sports injuries began to clear up with the gentle movements.

Professor Peter McKiernan
CHAIRMAN OF THE DEPARTMENT OF MANAGEMENT, UNIVERSITY OF ST ANDREWS, SCOTLAND

I have known Peter Chin Kean Choy for many years. He is a very capable person and organizer. He is an excellent teacher of T'ai-Chi Chi Kung.

Eileen Caddy
CO-FOUNDER OF THE FINDHORN FOUNDATION, SCOTLAND

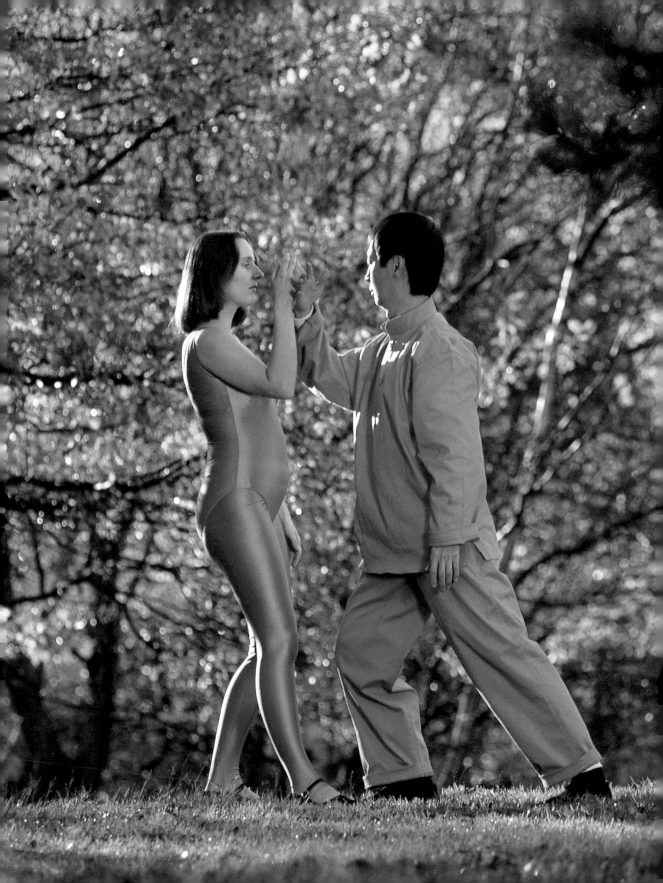

the realizing of the true **tao**

When Yin and Yang unite,
blissful feelings emerge,
the Tigress and Dragon embrace
in a T'ai-Chi Dance of Ecstasy.

Wu-Chi the matchmaker has
successfully blessed Yin and Yang.
Yin and Yang are intertwined into
a Happy Dream.

Effortlessly they approach the palace gates
and ascend into the Tao,
immersed in a Rainbow River of Chi.

Zhang Bo Duan
The Taoist Classics (eleventh century)

I dedicate this book to my parents, Chin Ket Leong and Yong Liu Keow, and to my teachers, relatives, friends and students for their love and support; and to the invisible wise ones who work silently behind the scenes bringing hope, healing and smiles to our most difficult moments.

t'ai chi chi kung

fifteen ways to a happier you

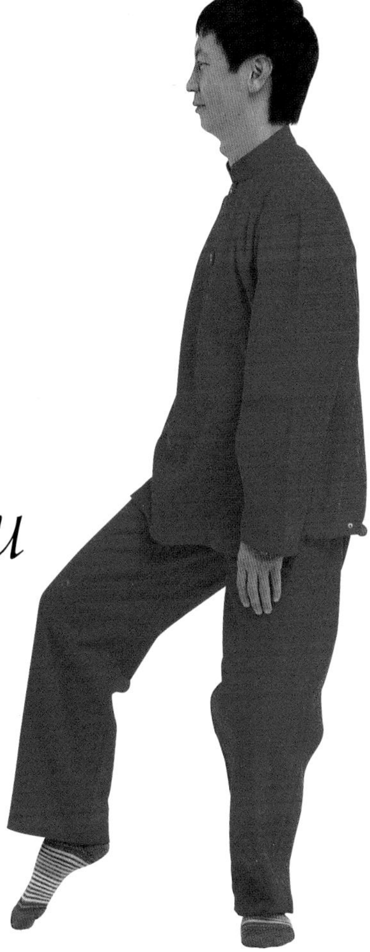

Peter Chin Kean Choy

THE OVERLOOK PRESS

WOODSTOCK AND NEW YORK

First published in the United States in 1999 by
The Overlook Press, Peter Mayer Publishers, Inc.
Lewis Hollow Road
Woodstock, New York 12498

ISBN: 0-87951-940-1

Photography by Christopher Cormack
Design by Geoff Hayes
Edited by Caroline Taggart

Special thanks to Dancia International of London for the loan of
dancewear. The photographs on pages 11 and 13 are by John Glover,
and those on pages 15, 17, 18, and 21 by Heather Angel.

A Cataloguing in Publication record for this title is available from
The Library of Congress.

1 3 5 7 9 8 6 4 2

A CIP catalog record of this book is available from The Library of
Congress.

Printed by Singapore by Kyodo Printing Co (S'pore) Pte Ltd

Important Note

*The information given in this book is intended for general guidance and is
not a substitute for individual diagnosis or treatment by a qualified
practitioner or medical doctor. If the reader is unwell, he/she is strongly
advised not to attempt self-treatment for any serious or long-term
complaint without consulting a medical doctor, a qualified
complementary health practitioner and/or a qualified FTT Certified Trainer.
Neither the author, the publishers nor The Rainbow T'ai-Chi Chi Kung
Centre can be held responsible for any adverse reaction to the
recommendations contained in this book, which are followed entirely at the
reader's own risk.*

There is a dimension where fountains of health and happiness await us,
a peaceful space where the light of love will heal the wounds in your heart,
where there are limitless smiles behind your smile.
It is already in you.
It is as real as the valves, arteries and veins flowing in you,
so why can't you get there then?
It is mainly because you are not slow enough to be in it.

Listen to the pauses
in between your breathing,
in between your heartbeats.
In the stillness,
you will feel the
Inner T'ai-chi Dance of Yin and Yang,
your every gestures a tingling of beauty and joy . . .

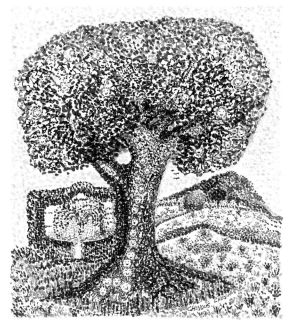

Melt into the Chi Energy of Health and Vitality,
and then, effortlessly,
you will discover more self-confidence.

It doesn't mean that there will be no problems hereafter
but you can see them as wonderful creative opportunities.

Abundance and health will
naturally flow through you and all around you.

Contents

Acknowledgements

I am grateful most of all to my unique teacher, U G Krishnamurti, who taught me T'ai-Chi Chi Kung of the Heart. It was from him that I learned to apply T'ai-Chi in my daily living. He gave no instructions on technique or form of exercise. Although some people did come to receive healings, his technique was not 'laying on of hands' or any kind of therapy that I knew of. It was simply in being. We sat, went for walks. We cooked, washed our dishes, swept the floor. This teaching of simply 'being in the T'ai-Chi energy' trained me to accept the unknown chi energy as an intelligent and wise friend. It helped me to find a heart-centred way to practise T'ai-Chi Chi Kung and discover who I really am and what my purpose is in this life.

I am also grateful to Master Huang (of Malaysia), who taught me the 'doing' part of the T'ai-Chi Yang Style Form and the Fundamental T'ai-Chi Chi Kung Exercises. Although only interested in the doing part of the T'ai-chi philosophy, Master Huang showed a childlike sense of humour, playfulness and humility. I would like to thank Dr T K Shih of the Chi Healing Centre (USA) and Dr Pang and the Chi Kung Teachers from the Zhineng Chi Kung Centre (China) for their indispensable training and advice in the art of chi healing. My work has also been inspired by the research of Professor Jou Tsung Hwa and Dr Yang Jwing Ming into the benefits of T'ai-Chi Chi Kung. My sincere thanks also go to Master Mantak Chia, who shared with me the love for all the ancient Taoist practices. All these people have helped me learn to find and create a balanced system of Rainbow T'ai-Chi Chi Kung Exercises and Principles.

Barry and Suzy Kaufman of the Option Institute (USA) and Peter and Eileen Caddy and Dorothy Maclean of the Findhorn Foundations (Scotland) have been positive sources of encouragement to my personal growth. Together with the eastern teachers, they helped me create a rainbow bridge of understanding in a western-world context. I am also immensely grateful to my father, Chin Ket Leong, who was a Chinese martial arts teacher and Chinese medical doctor. I am forever grateful for his lessons on discipline, patience, persistence and wisdom. To my mother, Yong Liu Keow, you will always be a living saint for me. I still don't know how you did it, being a mother, carrying seven of us around in your Volkswagen, and being a successful full-time school teacher. I now understand why the whole school turned out to say good-bye to you when you retired. They loved you. Thank you for inspiring me to keep on believing that the world does appreciate good teachers.

I am also deeply grateful to many people for coming at the ripe time and helping to produce the first two home-made versions of this book. Amongst them are Joe Hickey, Jason Davis and Corazon Wilkinson. In the second version, we went to the seaside and I want to send a big thank you to the Spirits of the Nature Elements: the sea, wind, sun, earth, trees and birds for their indispensable contribution to making this book truly a T'ai-chi experience. A very big affectionate thank you to Corazon Wilkinson for her meticulous and loving editing of the first edition of this book.

After that, this book found its way into the loving arms of Caroline Taggart and Kyle Cathie of Kyle Cathie Publishers. I want to thank Caroline for her amazing sense of intuition, trust, openness of mind to flow with whatever comes. I would also like to thank Christopher Cormack, the brilliant photographer of the colour photographs in the book. And Geoff Hayes for the fantastic design of the whole book. A special note of appreciation also goes to Michael, my tailor, who made, perfectly and according to my specifications, all the colourful T'ai-Chi clothes in this book. All the

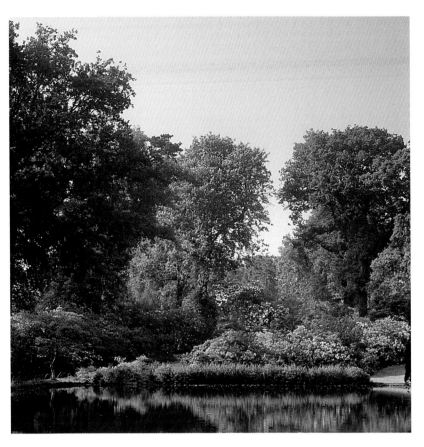

I have always admired you and am proud that you are my brother. I also want to thank Chan, Yap and Cornelius Bong for all the initial years of my searching. You were always there for me whenever I needed you. A very special thank-you to Francine Ismay, who has been not only an indispensable catalyst in helping to deepen my understanding of T'ai-Chi; she has also been a great source of inspiration to me through-out the writing of this book.

I would also like to thank all the thousands of T'ai-chi Chi Kung students over the past twenty-five years who have shared with me countless numbers of examples as to how they have successfully applied the T'ai-chi Chi Kung tools in their own lives. It would take more than a book this size to put down all your names and all your achievements, but this book would not be here without you. Thank you. You are the shimmering waves that often moved me to tears when I felt the beauty and radiance of your T'ai-Chi Chi Kung movements dancing in the hundreds of community halls throughout Europe, America and Asia – silently gliding across, boundless and free spirits of the chi. You are the unsung heroes and heroines who made real the nameless silent wise ones. How many times did you open your eyes and cry too when you saw that we were all flowing in this limitless sea of chi? You felt happy. Peaceful. Contented. Even if it was just for an instant, you and I realized we are truly at home to our tan-tien (literally translated as 'the Sea of Chi Energy'). Regardless of age, belief, colour, social status or profession, we are all swimming in this Ocean of Health and Happiness.

other tailors told me that it was impossible to complete the work in ten days and Michael did it in four! My thanks to Julie Timbrell, the lovely model demonstrating the Chi Kung exercises in this book. Julie has been studying T'ai-Chi Chi Kung with me for many years and recently graduated as a teacher.

There are many other people who have inspired me all these years. They have helped me carry on and they stuck by my side during the downs as well as the ups. Thank you Myriam Zink, Triune, Tao, Gael, Melchizedec, for teaching me unconditional love and sharing your joy for living. A heartfelt message to Tommy, my brother, who first inspired me to put down on paper my self-discoveries when we were young. My dearest brother Edward, I will never forget our teenage years when we spent hours every day meditating on the facts of life. One day you said, 'Shhh, listen, did you hear what the wind just said?' I said, 'No. What did it say?' And you said, 'The wind said, "I'm just passing by"' We have laughed so much during those times! And a big thank you goes to you, David and Helen, my older brother and sister, your efforts to keep on succeeding in your life in spite of difficult challenges will inspire me always. Thank you, Philip Ken, my brother, you are the best soccer player I ever knew. And I want the world to know you were the National Soccer Team Captain and you played in the First Division!

Preface

If you have read the verses on the first pages of this book, you may ask, 'Choy, can I really discover this inner fountain of health and rejuvenation?' And my reply is, 'Yes! I can show you how. Practise these fifteen Fundamental T'ai-Chi Chi Kung Exercises every day for one hundred days, and you will get there.'

Many people who have practised these fifteen exercises have told me how their lives have changed for the better. Not only has their health improved, but they have also had more vitality, enabling them successfully to undertake projects which they have been putting off for many years. The most effective way we have found to test whether the exercises were working or not lies in what students' relatives and friends say about them. Serious students who are making progress often report that their friends and relatives have made positive comments such as, 'You look younger and calmer – what have you been doing?'

What is their secret of youthfulness and rejuvenation? Answer: the quality time they put into their practice is investing chi energy into their lives. I was giving a class one morning recently and some people shared that they did not have time to practise. So, I said, 'Right, let us see. Which of the fifteen exercises makes you feel some chi energy? Which do you particularly enjoy doing during the class?' They showed me one exercise. I got them to go through it slowly, one step at a time. And then I asked, 'Did you feel the chi energy?' They nodded, yes. I asked, 'Now, how long did that take?' 'Three minutes?' they guessed. 'No,' I said, 'one minute!'

When people work very hard in an office or at home, at a desk or in front of a computer, they believe that they do not have any time. They have time for coffee breaks, they have time for a cigarette and a gossip, but no time for one minute of rejuvenating chi energy exercise?

But why is that one minute so important? Think of people saving in pension schemes or deposit accounts at the bank. After ten years, they have big smiles on their faces as they collect their investments, which have by that time accumulated a great deal in compound interest. Right?

Maybe one day, I will put a full-page advertisement in a national newspaper with the headline, 'Invest in the Chi Building Society'. In ten years, you will receive one million pounds of chi energy filled with health and rejuvenation. At the bottom of the advertisement I will put, 'For more details, phone yourself!' Look at those eighty- or ninety-year-old Chinese people who are as fit as eighteen- or nineteen-year-olds! My T'ai-Chi Master Huang is one of these people. What is their secret? Over the years, they have been saving a lot of chi credit units through the daily investment of a few minutes' practice. Through the practice they discover an inner door to a dimension of chi energy. It is like a visit to your favourite swimming pool or sauna/jacuzzi. Students often laugh when I tell them at the end of the class that I will see them at the local chi pub for a drink of chi energy or the jacu-chi!

Of course, when you start, you need support and time to learn the exercises well. This book provides a starting point. Go through it and pick any of the exercises to which you feel attracted. Experiment with it. It will give you a taste of what it could be like. You may start to feel some warm tingling sensations in your fingers or palms. Then, you might want to do more. We have a growing list of instructors in the UK – please write to the address on page 159 to find out if there is one in your area. We will also be holding courses outside the UK in the near future, and enquiries are always welcome. We often hold courses at the seaside – practising close to Nature enables you to learn faster too.

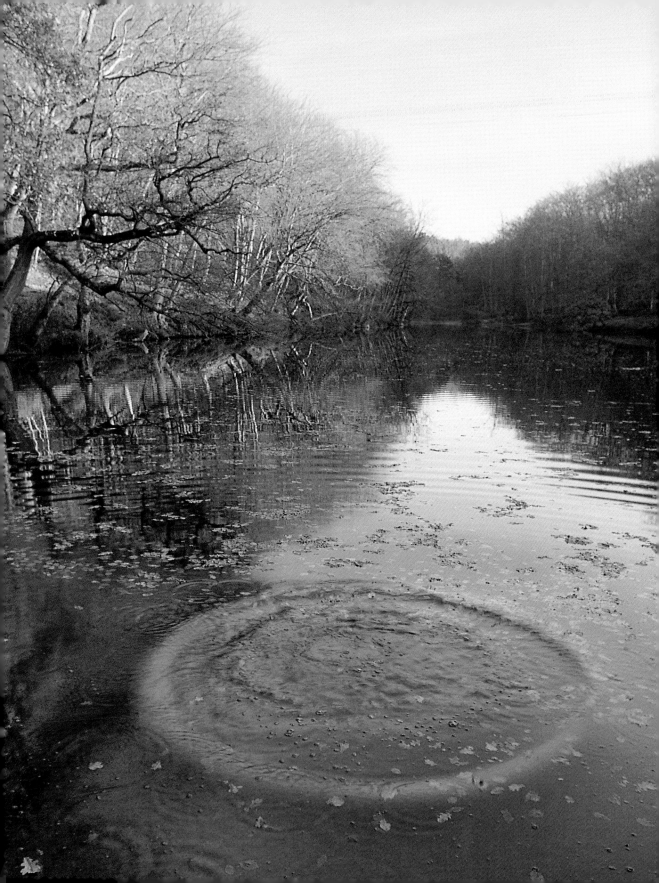

In the mean time, I have included a Five-Minute Workout rhythm for busy people. If you have more time, practise every day for 10–15 minutes. How much you get out of the exercises depends on how much you are willing to invest, multiplied a thousand fold in terms of greater health and rejuvenation.

So, what do I hope you will gain from this book?

In addition to the benefit I know you will derive from these exercises, I believe that this book might show you the possibility of discovering who you really are. That is why the homework sections are equally as important as the exercises themselves. I would like you to use the homework 'to guide yourself home to your naturally abundant source of chi'. I mean this in a creative, down-to-earth way as well as on an emotional, intuitive and rational level.

When the ancient Taoists explained that there were acupuncture points called 'Bubbling Well' on the underside of your feet, and that longevity could be attained by learning to breathe from the feet, were they speaking metaphorically? Here lies another secret of how to discover the inner fountain of youth and rejuvenation – it is right under your feet.

I hope that by using this book you will learn to think on your feet and 'under-stand' the way home to who you really are. You are a being of energy. May your feet guide you home to your tan-tien, the chi energy centre of your being. May Nature's Dance of Chi Energy truly help you to nourish your organs. Invest in

healthy organs. Understand that your organs need a touch of kindness, compassion and gentleness from your heart, and that if they receive this they will give you a long and healthy life. You would stretch out and touch a man who had fallen by the roadside, and give compassion, kindness and gentleness if he was hurt, wouldn't you? Why not do the same for your organs? Many of the Chi Kung exercises in this book give you the opportunity to do this.

The realistic way to achieve longevity and good health in the long term is surely to build a loving relationship with your body. In T'ai-Chi Chi Kung, you can literally dance your way into an inner fountain of rejuvenating energy inside and outside your body. At the end of a recent class, someone shared, 'I feel stoned, except that there are no side effects and it feels so natural and effortless.' You are always surrounded by cosmic chi energy. You only have to slow down your mind to rediscover this fact.

I have found that the Rainbow T'ai-Chi Chi Kung exercises and principles are readily accepted by people from many different religious backgrounds. I have had Buddhists, Christians and Muslims in my classes. A nun even shared with me how she found the movements to be like 'prayer in motion'. Another student said, 'It is like poetry in motion.' A Buddhist recently shared how she was able to use the exercises and principles to help accelerate the healing of her lower back pain.

I would also like to give you another perspective on why I believe anyone, whether oriental or occidental, can

discover this inner fountain of rejuvenating energy. I run classes at the Rainbow T'ai-Chi Chi Kung Centre, and you may have noticed that the exercises in this book are 'coded' according to the colours of the rainbow. Many people ask, 'Why "Rainbow"?' Some years ago, a trainee asked me what I got out of the course I was running for future teachers of T'ai-Chi Chi Kung. I replied that the course unfolded and synthesized seven rainbow aspects in my life. Each of the rainbow colours represents a blending of Yin and Yang qualities (please refer to the Seventh Fundamental T'ai-Chi Exercise/Principle, page 70, for more explanation of this).

As the people who come into the training programme with their multi-coloured talents and qualities grow and feel more empowered in themselves, I see them as rainbow reflections of myself. The concept of Rainbow T'ai-Chi Chi Kung is also connected to the Four Seasons Chi Kung (see the exercises on pages 100–111), especially when you practise them out of doors in front of a sunrise. See the sparkling jewel-like kaleidoscope of brilliant rainbow lights shining towards you from the dewdrops.

Countless times, when we have practised this sequence of exercises outside, just after it has been raining, the sun has shone through and we have seen double, sometimes triple rainbows in the sky above us. We dance in between the Yin/water and Yang/warmth of the rain and sun to bring Rainbow T'ai-Chi Chi Kung to the earth. Pure, fresh, natural chi will flow through you like an invisible fountain, awakening every cell in

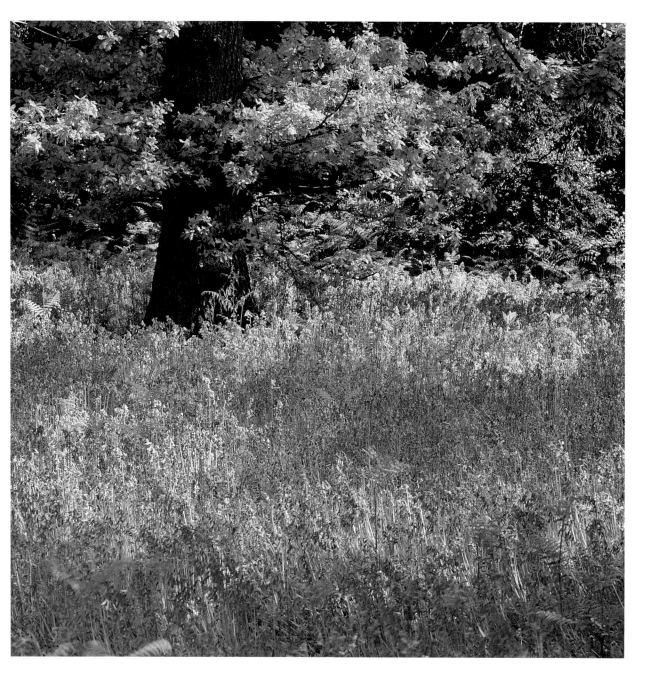

your whole being to the fact that they too come from pure natural chi. At the end of such a morning's practice, I often ask everyone to find a blade of grass with some rainbow dewdrops and pluck it gently to share it with someone. You can imagine the giggles that follow, as people attempt to put these tiny blades close to their partners' mouths! People often share that this part of their workshop experience is one of the most memorable – like drinking in tingling chi first thing in the morning. A cup of chi a day keeps you healthy all day! Some ancient T'ai-Chi Chi Kung practitioners have spoken poetically about discovering the secrets of youth and rejuvenation through the absorption of the 'first rays of sunlight while dancing on the dewdrops in the early morning'.

Another thing you may have noticed is that the subtitle of the book is not 'Fifteen Ways to a Happy You' but 'Fifteen Ways to a *Happier* You'. I believe there is already a happy being filled with pure rejuvenating chi within you – it is just waiting for you to discover it. Many great T'ai-Chi Masters, like Professor Cheng Man-Ching, speak of a baby learning to walk as the best example of a T'ai-Chi practitioner. When you watch a baby going from the crawling stage to learning how to walk, you will notice that the child does not judge his crawling as 'good crawling' or 'bad crawling'. Neither is he motivating himself to learn to walk by blaming crawling as a bad experience. His face is serene and happy when he is crawling.

In the same way, for the child or adult learning T'ai-Chi Chi Kung, the art of growing can be a non-judgmental process of learning how to find balance within situations of imbalance. We can rediscover this pure chi energy within ourselves because we are all born with it.

Is it possible to discover that you are truly a naturally happy and relaxed person and that you can effortlessly let go of your unhappy and stressful ways of thinking and acting? The exercises and principles in this book are aimed at reminding you of the way home to this naturally happy being and also at taking you one step further. You can experience it with your physical body. Your body will find it easier to do well in other sports and generally to improve all areas of your life. The more relaxed, effortless

and confident you are, the more 'goodies' you will be able to receive from life.

You can experience the fountain of rejuvenation when you feel the chi literally purifying and circulating through your body's blood vessels, bringing fresh and revitalizing new energy to every cell of your whole being. You spend it again as you go about your daily chores, and then you use the exercises and principles to 'recharge your inner batteries', as one student recently said to me.

After learning the fifteen Fundamental T'ai-Chi and Chi Kung exercises, you may ask, 'Where do I go from here?' The ancients believed that the study of chi energy had many branches. The seven Chi Kung exercises in this book are like the roots of a tree and the eight Fundamental T'ai-Chi exercises are like the lower part of the trunk. The thirty-seven step Yang-style T'ai-Chi – taught in many books and evening classes – is like the upper part of the trunk and branches which flows and dances with the elements of Nature. Other advanced studies include the Foundation T'ai-Chi Chi Kung one-year training programme (FTT), Foundation Teacher Trainers for FTT (F3T), the Taoist Trilogue Communication Intensive, Fusion of the Five Elements of Nature (for improving the health of your internal organs), Kan and Li (an inner art of steaming and purification for rejuvenating your body), Bone Marrow Chi Kung (a meditative exercise to promote longevity) and Zhineng Chi Kung (Cosmic Chi Kung exercises for improving your chi healing abilities). To help you learn more effectively, we also have

some videos and music cassettes, which will be especially useful if you do not yet have an instructor nearby. They will not compensate for the absence of a Rainbow T'ai-Chi Chi Kung teacher, but they are the next best thing. There are more details about these at the end of the book.

I believe that one day people will be able to experience chi energy as an absolutely normal phenomenon and that it will be as accepted as such. Until that day comes, I will carry on working to help more people become aware of the value and benefit of this practice.

I hope you enjoy this book as much as I have enjoyed writing it. Please do write to me and share experiences about how you have used the exercises.

Although I do encourage everyone using this book to share it with others, I hope that that will not be taken as permission to teach the exercises and earn an income from so doing. It takes a long training programme to make good teachers. Like bakers who are proud of the loaves they make, we do not want to send out half-baked bread, do we? So, by all means, experiment with the exercises and have fun with them. But if you are serious about learning to be an instructor, write to me for information about training programmes.

May limitless chi filled with joy, health and vitality continue to flow in your life and overflow to touch everyone around you.

PETER CHIN KEAN CHOY

Introduction

The Taoist way is the way of Nature
As far back as 2690 BC, according to Chinese historians, before the era of acupuncture, Buddhism and martial arts, the study of chi was embodied in a Chinese natural science called Tao – the Way of Nature. Chinese physicians applied their understanding of Nature to the maintenance of health and the cure of illness. They studied the balance of the opposite forces in Nature, which they called Yin and Yang and which they saw in all sorts of aspects – shadow and light, negative and positive, masculine and feminine, hard and soft, summer and winter, fire and water, spring and autumn, and wood and metal. Through chi meditation and exercises the Taoists also discovered chi energy links with the internal organs.

The chi exercises were about the practice of harmonizing Nature's five elements (water, earth, air, wood and metal), the three chi treasures of Nature (earth chi, human chi and heavenly chi) and the four seasons (spring, summer, autumn and winter). The underlying purpose was and is to learn how to generate, conserve and channel chi for health and longevity.

What exactly is chi?
For readers unfamiliar with the term, chi is a Chinese word meaning 'intrinsic energy'. In India, the yogis call it 'prana'. According to all teachers of the ancient arts of T'ai-Chi and Chi Kung, chi energy can be experienced by balancing the Yin/ feminine/receptive and Yang/ masculine/emissive principles within your life. Many alternative therapists call this the life force. There are many different ways in which you can channel this life force to achieve a balanced state of health, rejuvenation and harmony. You can practise balancing your energies purely on one level or a mixture of different levels – physical, mental or emotional.

On the physical level, for example, you could use medication, diet, sleeping patterns, change of job or relationship to find a better balance of Yin and Yang in your lifestyle. You

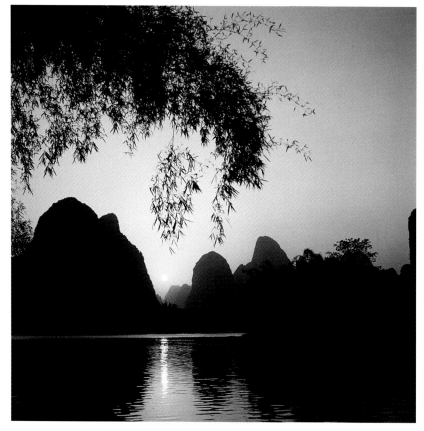

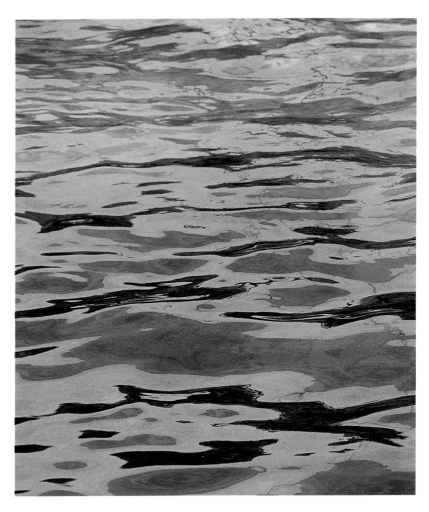

believe that each group is unique and doing the best it can based on its own experiences, structures, principles and disciplines. I have been trained to work with the heart centre first. I prefer to consider it as dynamic, moving energy located around the chest rather than as a specific physical location. It has been known as the middle tan-tien (and tan-tien is Chinese for 'sea of energy'), so asking where the heart centre lies is a bit like asking where is the centre of the sea.

The heart centre has also been called 'a pool of chi energy'. How do we experience it? We cannot see it, but we can feel it as a warm, glowing and tingling sensation. Through the practice of the exercises in this book, especially the Third Fundamental T'ai-Chi Exercise (page 40) and the First Chi Kung Exercise (page 86), you will learn about the benefits of heart-beat listening and learning to flow with the heart meridian energy. You will discover that the heart centre is not simply a metaphor but a very physical experience. After many years of practising the Four Seasons Chi Kung Exercise (see page 100), you may also experience being inside your arteries (carrying Yin/nurturing blood) and veins (carrying Yang/ spent blood) and feeling the power of ten thousand oceans circulating through your body. Chinese medical practitioners believe that the heart is the governor of all inner flow of chi energy. This is another reason why we encourage students to practise this first step before starting the physical exercises.

might also go to a counsellor or therapist to help you find a more balanced perspective about some emotional issues. When you feel the need to talk about some pressing emotional issues, this 'need to share' is the Yang principle. (You will notice throughout this book that I often use the word 'share' when someone is talking about their experiences or response to the exercises.) The presence of a receptive person listening helps you find a balance with the Yin principle.

An overworked person is too Yang and will feel better when he or she relaxes (Yin). Someone who is too Yin in mental attitude, in the sense of being too self-conscious, analytical and introverted, might feel more balance if he did some kind of physical activity that helped him to unwind and become more confident. When you balance the Yin and Yang aspects of your life, you will feel new energy, better health and more enthusiasm in your life.

The heart centre, tan-tien centre and eyes/Yin-tang centre
Many therapeutic groups work with different health-generating energies, moving towards the same goals. I

So, once you have contacted the heart centre or middle tan-tien, you learn to work with the lower tan-tien or belly centre. You learn to co-ordinate your upper and lower limbs from this centre. You learn to absorb chi energy into this centre and direct the chi to be stored in your internal organs for good health and rejuvenation. Some people believe that the tan-tien is 5cm (2in) below the navel, while others believe it is at the centre of the navel. But it is important to remember that we are once again speaking about the tan-tien as a 'sea of energy'. Yes, it is in the navel centre, and yes, it is also around the navel centre. It is a powerful flowing force of vitality which gives you tremendous stamina as well as providing a 'gut feeling' of confidence to make clear and balanced decisions. How do you learn balance? For example, in the Second and Sixth Fundamental T'ai-Chi exercises (see pages 30 and 64), you learn to co-ordinate your upper and lower limbs as well as work on an emotional and heart tan-tien level to bring more balance, harmony and wisdom back into your daily life.

From the heart and belly centres, we connect chi energy to the yin-tang upper tan-tien centre between the eyes. This pool of energy is linked to our thinking and understanding. The balancing of this mental chi energy is important in the study of T'ai-Chi Chi Kung. It enables us to under-stand logically, visually and cognitively what we experience.

What is T'ai-Chi Chi Kung?
Chi exercises fall into two main categories – Chi Kung and T'ai-Chi. The study of the secrets of rejuvenation and healing is called Chi Kung. The ancient Chinese Chi Kung Masters showed tremendous patience in studying the connection

between the Way of Nature (the Tao) and chi energy. This is why Chi Kung (sometimes written as Qi Gong) is defined by Chinese scholars as 'the study of chi energy'. It has been wrongly interpreted as a set of breathing exercises. Most traditional Chi Kung teachers emphasize that breathing must be normal. Chi energy is experienced in the air element during normal breathing when you relax during the movements. You come to understand that chi already exists in normal breathing and see it as a regular part of your life. Chi Kung experts do use a combination of chi energy, emotional calm, breath control, sound and physical movement to help others in healing sessions.

The element of water motivated early practitioners to formulate their understanding of T'ai-Chi, which means 'the river of energy which unites Yin and Yang into a dance and flows into the sea of energy (tan-tien)'. The practice of T'ai-Chi exercises opens up the gates and meridian channels of energy in the body, helps relax the muscles and ligaments, and regulates the blood circulation. The Chi Kung exercises help to generate, channel, conserve, store and direct the energy into the body to achieve optimum health.

The importance of cognitive skills training
Today's scientists have proved that all matter is made up of millions upon millions of energy particles. For them this is a fact, but can they experience it with their emotions? I have been fortunate enough to meet some scientists who came to learn with me and they have proved to themselves that yes, they can melt

into pure limitless energy in their physical movements. So, with their emotion, thinking and physical actions, they can actually verify the scientific principle that all matter is made up of energy! I believe that one of the greatest gifts of the Taoist science is to add a cognitive heart/body/mind/spirit approach to occidental scientific discoveries.

However, most people who have been educated to think in a recognitive way may find it difficult to grasp this natural cognitive way of learning. The recognitive way is to recognize things and experiences with the mind rather than to perceive them directly first hand. It is as if you went to buy a new car and somehow ended up with a used, second-hand car. In the cognitive approach your senses see something in a new and fresh way; in the recognitive they refer back to a past associated experience in order to understand what they are experiencing now.

When you are doing any new kind of activity, whether learning T'ai-Chi or learning to play a musical instrument, your mind sometimes seems to observe the action and make critical comments such as 'I have never been any good at this sort of thing'. This is not simply lack of self-confidence or build-up of stress. This inherent fact about learning processes has to do with where the learner is. You need to understand not just the instrument but also the teacher and what is expected of you. When you can finally overcome the recognitive feeling of self-consciousness, something clicks. You feel a sense of flowing oneness with the activity. Another example is to imagine yourself standing in front of a group of people, making a speech or singing a song. Children's cognitive faculties are more predominant and they can often do this sort of thing effortlessly. An adult who has recognitive experiences of fearing the unknown or of making a fool of him/herself will find this much more difficult and embarrassing.

So, how do you acquire the cognitive approach to learning?

In terms of T'ai-Chi, if you are a total beginner, this is good news! Your sense of openness and curiosity is like the mind of a child. You feel one with the T'ai-Chi Chi Kung movements.

Most people who have done some years of practice can feel a sense of oneness, especially if they practise out of doors. You can feel a sense of oneness with trees in the First Chi Kung Exercise (see page 86). In the Four Seasons Chi Kung (page 100), you can feel the cycle of the four seasons flowing into your whole being. In the Sixth Fundamental T'ai-Chi Exercise (page 64), you can feel like a seagull. The natural harmonization of these exercises with visual correspondences is effortless.

The cognitive nature of learning can be traced to how the Chinese language was created. The Han Dynasty lexicographer Xu Shen, who lived from 30 to 124 AD, found that 'natural image shapes' became 'Chinese picture characters'. For example, the Chinese character for water was literally like a flowing river! The character for man was a drawing of a man and for woman a woman of humble character! This reveals a relationship between the emotion, thinking and physical nature of the ancient Taoists – their direct or cognitive way of perceiving life and their recognitive way of communicating that perception was truly pure and simple.

The benefits of the cognitive approach

On the emotional level, what does it mean to use the cognitive attitude in communicating with other people? It means you are letting go of all previous recognitive perceptions of the other person you are talking to and you really want to hear what that other person is saying, without prejudging or assuming. You want a direct perception of the other person's point of view. You are using the T'ai-Chi yielding principle of Investment in Loss (as written in the T'ai-Chi Classics) to neutralize reactive feelings (that is, feelings coming from yourself first) before responding to someone else. This helps you to slow down and really listen to the other person. The other person will begin to feel that you are genuinely doing your best to understand what he or she is saying. Then you can truly feel at ease and the other person feels comfortable with you, too. Together, you learn to co-operate rather than compete with each other to resolve issues.

On the physical level, when you are drawing, painting, sketching, gardening, cooking, playing music, etc., your cognitive approach enables you to perceive directly the object or subject you are interested in. You see it as it is, without any preconceived ideas. You are melting into the scenery, the paints, brushes and canvas. You produce a marvellous dish that surprises everyone because you flowed with the recipe, the kitchen and the people you were cooking for. You may also have added your own magical touch to the recipe. If you are a gardener you feel a rhythmic sense of harmony with the seedling plants, the muck and the weather.

On the mental level, you can practise directly perceiving a thought or image, as well as the spaces between thoughts. You can use the cognitive/receptive attitude of T'ai-Chi to 'make friends' with your mind. You will learn how to do this as you work through the exercises. Many old schools of thought promote the idea that the mind needs to be trained, to be tamed like a wild monkey and taught how to concentrate. However, when your mind has more accepting space within the consciousness, it naturally brings about order, like a tree effortlessly stretching its trunk, branches, twigs, leaves and fruits.

On a spiritual level, you do not judge critically should you see visions and experience ecstatic states of consciousness. Through direct perception, you become one with the vision. You also give yourself permission to come out of it and to find balance with your emotional, mental and physical aspects.

The heart/body/mind/spirit way to encourage learning

The heart/body/mind/spirit approach to T'ai-Chi Chi Kung is to encourage you to feel a sense of total oneness with whatever you are focusing on – the cognitive approach.

This enables you truly to love, enjoy and understand what you are doing, and really to hear what your teacher is saying and wants you to do. So, the first step is bringing your heart – not your mind – into the scene.

When the physical body enjoys the learning process, naturally every action feels more fluid and effortless. The mind then records the action as an effortless and enjoyable activity. What follows are natural awakenings of intuitive and rational insights into whatever you are doing.
So, how do you apply this heart/body/mind/spirit learning process?

This is what this book can do for you. There are fifteen exercises to get your mind to slow down and relearn how to live a more fulfilling and healthier life. For example, in the Third Fundamental T'ai-Chi Exercise (see page 40), you learn about heart-beat listening. This can help you slow down and learn to listen cognitively; this in turn will help you form a strong basis for learning about chi healing. To give another example, you can bring more balance into your life by learning the heart exercise in the Second Fundamental T'ai-Chi Exercise (page 30).

The practice of the heart/body/ mind/spirit approach to T'ai-Chi and Chi Kung learning started for me when I was in primary school. I was interested in the way chi energy works within our minds. The school teachers were not very impressed! I recall a classmate saying he had a headache and I asked, 'Where is it? Is it always at a fixed point in your head or does it move?' My friend said, 'Yes, it is moving over to here . . .' And I said, 'What happens if you stay with it, like watching a snake moving around?' 'My headache, it is gone!' my friend exclaimed in surprise. And I whispered, 'Now, can you feel the energy moving in your body?' We were in a biology class, learning about the different parts of the body. The teacher reprimanded me for not paying attention. Little did she realize that I really was paying attention, in more depth than she could have expected.

Over the years since then, I have gone in search of teachers to deepen my understanding and knowledge of chi healing. After conducting thousands of successful chi healings on myself and on others, I decided to help train other people. Over the years, my students have produced wonderful results. The chi healing section in this book (page 136) is a fresh glimpse into how people have used the T'ai-Chi Chi Kung principles to facilitate their self-healing processes, as well as a brief report on our research into the benefits of chi healings conducted with more than a hundred people.

T'ai-Chi Chi Kung for children
Now, coming back to education. Did you know that the root meaning lies in the Latin word *educere* – to lead out? Back in school, I did not feel that I was being led out in my understanding about the energy in my body. I was given a lot of information to memorize and this had to do more with passing tests than with me. So, I promised myself that when I grew up, I would help people grow through rediscovering life's abundant energies, which are already within them.

This is why I have included a special section on T'ai-Chi Chi Kung for children (page 117), to help them learn how to relax and discover a sense of harmony in their body movements. Children are the leaders of our future. If they are able to get more in touch with chi energy in a balanced way, perhaps the dream of a more balanced and healthier humanity might not be too far off. Children need encouragement if they are to remember their natural vital force.

Daily applications of T'ai-Chi Chi Kung
Although T'ai-Chi Masters often taught that T'ai-Chi Chi Kung was a system of health and rejuvenation and that the martial arts aspect was merely an extension of the philosophy of the Tao, we seem to have made little progress in terms of applying the principles to improving students' lives on a day-to-day basis. So, the chapters on practising T'ai-Chi Chi Kung in your daily life (page 112) and the Five-Minute T'ai-Chi Chi Kung Workout (page 132) emphasize the importance of an integrated system of education that becomes an integral part of your daily life.

If education is about growing and learning, this is it. It is in the midst of our daily life that we need the vital force. If you bend over to carry something heavy, it is at that moment you need energy. Not later, when you go to a class. And what happens if your car breaks down? You need extra energy to push it to the side of the road – now! Your floor needs sweeping or vacuuming. If you do it with chi energy, it is enjoyable; if not, it's drudgery. T'ai-Chi Chi Kung can help educate people to maximize the vital force so that they can do physical work with ease.

Tao of Rainbow T'ai-Chi Chi Kung
Another favourite topic for the stressed-out modern man is money. The chapter on the Tao of Rainbow T'ai-Chi Chi Kung (page 142) is about how to make friends with your inner self and money. Through the practical use and understanding of this ancient science of colours and their corresponding qualities, we can attract health and prosperity to our lives. I hope that, after working through the chapter, you will feel the stresses in that part of your daily life lessened, if not transformed into joy and lightness.

The Foundation T'ai-Chi Chi Kung (FTT) Training Course
This gives me even more impetus to highlight the importance of T'ai-Chi Chi Kung. And this is not only my point of view. In the last chapter – The Foundation T'ai-Chi Chi Kung (FTT) Training Course (page 148) – you will read about the experiences of other teacher trainees and share their love and enthusiasm for this ancient art. The FTT is about people learning to use the Fifteen Fundamental T'ai-Chi Chi Kung Exercises/Principles as tools for personal growth. Today, there are very few qualified instructors available. I get many calls and letters from different associations asking for instructors and we do not have enough to go around. It takes many years of serious study truly to absorb the teachings. If you do not know of a qualified instructor locally and you want to bring T'ai-Chi Chi Kung to your area, let me know. If we do not have an instructor, I might ask you if you would like to apply to train as one!

Even after thousands of years, the study and practice of chi energy exercises continues to help people live a better life. The ancient Chinese teachers were right – there is a timeless value to the teachings of T'ai-Chi Chi Kung.

A note on the illustrations

The physical reality of ideas

My illustrations are usually based on physical, tangible objects. Not only have I attempted to find metaphors for the many abstract philosophical ideas expressed in this book, but I have found that the process of looking is also an experience of awakening. To benefit from this feature of the book, it is important that you slow down your mind and look with your heart. But what are you looking for?

Let me give you an example. In the introductory pages to this book, you will see an illustration of a fountain with a tree beside it. (This illustration and the poem it accompanies connect to the Eighth Fundamental T'ai-Chi experience of the inner fountain, see page 74.) This fountain and this tree actually existed. They were in front of the house in southern France where I lived for many years. I was inspired to learn that there were seven underground streams meeting under this fountain. In the olden days people used to bathe in it, and some came from long distances to collect water from it. Many claimed to be healed by drinking the water. So, when I show you an illustration of this fountain, there is a connection between the physical, emotional, mental and spiritual levels.

Why the dots and dotted lines?

These dots represent how I have experienced chi energy in all matter. They are like the atoms, molecules, ions, protons and neutrons of the fountain and the tree. Just as when we watch television we see the sum total of many thousands of pixels coming together to form pictures, so these tiny particles of chi energy form pictures too. I am also interested in awakening in the observer an awareness of the spaces between the dots and the lines. These spaces enable your mind to slow down, to re-examine what you see. Our minds become so familiar with the form, the lines, the dots, that that familiarity temporarily numbs the mind, turning it off from the chi energy. The crystallization of thought structure traps the chi in form and colour; sensations such as 'That's nice, that's not nice' take over and all the freshness of perception goes out the window. The mind comes alive again when you train it to look at spaces. Given sufficient space and time to be in stillness, it sees clearly, thinks rationally and acts wisely.

Chi energy and the physical body

There has been a lot of reliable research into reports of near-death experiences by thousands of people otherwise unknown to each other. This surely proves the belief that we are made up of energy and can retain consciousness of this when the body has been declared medically dead. The heart and brain have stopped functioning. Logically, you cannot be floating above the operating table or going through a tunnel and meeting light presences on the other side. You are supposed to be dead! The experiences of many of these people remind me of the hundreds of testimonials I have heard from practitioners of T'ai-Chi Chi Kung. They too sometimes feel that when they are doing the meditative exercises, they go through an inner tunnel and meet light presences. The difference is that they did not have to have a near-death experience!

Why the smiling, childlike faces in the drawings?

The Taoist Masters with whom I learned taught me that smiling energy is important to the harmonious flow of chi and that we need it to maintain the health of our organs. One of them, Dr T K Shih, goes so far as to say that smiling energy and chi energy are one and the same in chi healing. And even before I heard this from my Masters, I had my own strange experience of smiling presences.

In 1972, during my early years of T'ai-Chi Chi Kung training, I was in my room with Blackie, my dog, when a Fountain of Joy suddenly appeared in front of me. This was not a visualization exercise, nor was I taking any drugs – it simply appeared. It was like looking into limitless layers and layers of smiles. Over the years I have brought myself and thousands of others into this inner joyous healing lake and fountains where the bubbling chi energy has healed wounds and hurts. You feel your whole being bathed in waves of tingling beauty and joy. How do you know this is real and not just my imagination? That is what the book and the illustrations are all about. You need only to slow down and bring your heart, body, mind and spirit to touch and see this chi energy. It is not some kind of airy-fairy experience – as you will see as you go through the book, you can actually apply it to your daily life and see tremendous creative changes.

So, the way I experience this dimension is that there are smiling light beings who live there! They are inside us, too. Every time you light up when you see a baby smile its purest, innocent smile at you, it reminds you of your own inner spark. This sparkling essence belongs to the dimension of the smiling light beings. We seem to lose this spark when our minds and emotions are filled with worries, stresses, hurts and aches.

I hope, through my illustrations, to remind you that you have these natural sparks in you still. Try counting how many smiling faces you see on the tree beside the fountain at the front of the book, and write and tell me. You get a prize if it is the right answer!

This unique, beautiful and happy being inside you wakes up and smiles when someone else out there says, 'Hi' with a smile. Of course, if you like, you can go back to your conditioned mind, which says, 'Go away, I don't trust you. I want to be miserable and I will be a miser with my smiles. I am not able to smile back at you. I have no good news.' You could go on living that way for the next thirty years with organs that complain that you never take care of them and give them any smiles, strokes or appreciation.

You could smile for no particular reason. Or you could smile for a reason. Compare the two. Which one is like the baby's smile? When you practise your rainbow T'ai-Chi Chi Kung with me, you will start to realize that not only are there smiles, but there are Smiles. There are smiles of a peaceful feeling inside you, when you are so still that you could sit in the same spot for all eternity.

There are smiles that feel beautiful inside you because you feel your heart opening like a flower and every little movement around your heart feels so excruciatingly beautiful! There are smiles that make you cry because it is so lovely to see such a smile coming from within you. There are smiles that are like beams shining out from you. You see these smiles on children's faces when they have not seen you for some time and they have missed you. There are smiles that come after you have laughed so hard that your stomach aches and you want the person who is making you laugh to stop. There are smiles that bubble up like an uncontrollable and illogical

giggle when you sit around very, very serious people putting their heads together to consider an issue that is really quite simple.

Now, next time you see a tree – or any physical object – you may see it differently. Your mind may sense it more as an energy presence which is alive, rather than as a crystallized, more or less static object. Or you may respond differently to your body, your internal organs. How do you interact with your body? Do you treat it as a being of energy, or like a car to be sent to the garage for repairs when something is wrong with it? Do you give yourself space to feel what kind of a relationship you have with your body? Do you give it smiles of gratitude even when there is nothing wrong?

The power of genuine smiles of gratitude can really lighten up your body's relationship with you and vice versa. It is my hope that the smiling little beings I have drawn in this book will help you get back to your naturally happy self and make you even happier!

The fifteen fundamental T'ai-chi Chi Kung exercises

General guidelines

There are two ways to use this book. One is to flip through it and try out any of the exercises that appeal to you. Have a taste of it. The other way is to go through it systematically, working through the exercises one by one. If you are a complete beginner, you should try to practise for 10–15 minutes each morning and 10–15 minutes each evening. It will take you about a week to learn the physical, technical aspects of each exercise, and at least another week to apply the 'homework' section. Some of the homeworks will take longer, as you need to plan and prepare the assignment.

If you have some background in bodywork, such as yoga, martial arts or relaxation exercise, you may want to increase each session to 30 minutes or an hour, in order to deepen your experiences and benefit more from the exercises. It is a bit like learning to swim – once you enjoy swimming, the time vanishes!

Checklist for the exercises

Before you start the exercises, read through these guidelines and bear them in mind as you practise. You will feel more comfortable and the chi energy will flow more readily.

Feet

1 Stand with your feet apart, about the width of your shoulders.
2 Keep your feet parallel to one another.
3 When you move, keep most of your weight on one foot only.
4 Allow the change of weight in your feet be slow and gradual.
5 Sink all your weight down along your spine and down to the feet, like a tree anchoring its roots.

Knees

6 Keep your knees slightly bent, so that they are over your toes.

Waist

7 Co-ordinate your elbow movements from the waist.
8 Co-ordinate your wrists and fingers from your elbows connected to your waist.
9 Hold your spine and head vertical and move in harmony with your waist.

Hands

10 Move your palms in the air as leaves on a tree sway in response to the slightest pressure, even when a feather alights on them.
11 Keep your hands slightly curved, like a rainbow.

Shoulders

12 Relax and open up your shoulders.

Listening

13 Listen to your heartbeats and to the pauses in between.
14 Listen to the breathing in your belly and to the pauses in between.

Head

15 Keep your head upright, as if you were a puppet being pulled gently from above by the scalp.
16 Relax your facial muscles and jaw.

Breathing

17 Breathe slowly and deeply, like the wind passing through a tunnel, inhaling as your arms rise and/or extend outwardly, exhaling as your arms return and/or descend.

Recording your inspirations

18 After exercising, write down any inspiring insights, using T'ai-Chi as a mirroring experience.

☯ First T'ai-Chi Exercise/Principle

Find your peaceful and happy self by releasing your role plays

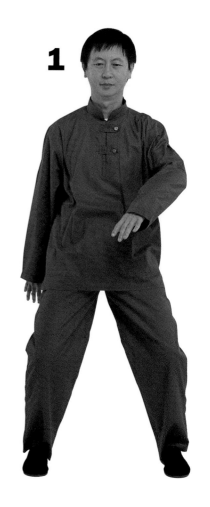

When to practise
This exercise is useful when you feel overburdened by responsibilities.

Best time to practise
In the evening when you come back from work or whenever you need it.

Tao of Violet Lessons
Learn to let go and allow more peaceful and pure healing energy to flow into your life.

1 Starting from the centre of your waist, swing your left arm up above your head, as far as it will go.

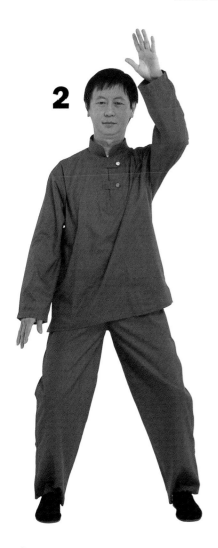

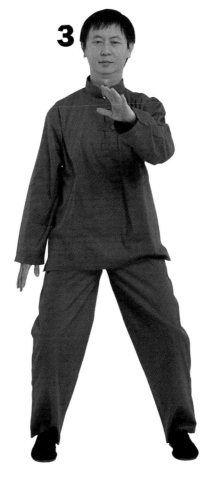

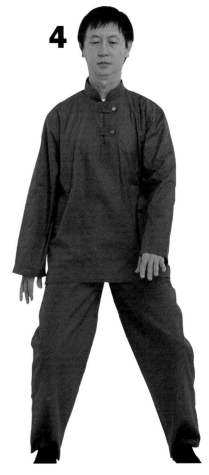

2 Point your fingertips upwards. Let your elbow take the weight of your arm. At the same time let your left arm swing forward and back by your side.

(Optional addition: At this point in the exercise you can also say aloud the words, 'I release all my . . . (pause).'

3 Suddenly, let your arm drop. (Optional addition: At this point you can also say aloud the corresponding words, '. . . role plays now!')

Do this, swinging from your waist for your right arm too. This exercise is about letting go of the tensions on your shoulders. When you feel responsible, you feel you are 'shouldering' responsibilities, as if you were wearing a jacket with the shoulders padded with tension.

4 Return to the original position and do the same with your right hand.

Note: You can also do this exercise in a slower and more meditative, Yin-like rhythm.

Letting go

When you feel heavy,
find it difficult to let go,
tried to escape, doing this, doing that,
running here, running there,
and now, trying to let go,
Are they both not from the same feeling,
a cry of frustration from deep within?

'What can I do?' you feel like screaming.
Okay, let's go for a walk.
Swing your hands,
throw your arm up,
Even now, you may beat yourself:
'Ahhh, I wish I hadn't done that!'
Round and round, like a merry-go-
round; finally, a feeling of 'I don't know
what to do!'
Feeling lost and nothing else to hold on
to?
Waves and waves of tears have come and
gone,
A great feeling of emptiness is all you've
got.

The last time you were happy seems such
a long time ago,
and now, you have no other choice but
sit back, lie back.
What else can you do?
Why not let the earth teach you,
this planet floating in outer space,
a sea of nothingness awaiting you,
so natural to ease into.

Have you finally slowed down?

Come and feel this feeling in your belly
centre.
Spirals coming and going,
Something you could spend your whole
life learning about,
no words, not even one single thought,
just breathe.

Feels good, doesn't it?

You don't need drugs, cigarettes, coffee.
Relax into the unknown – a silent friend,
no more fear, no more running away,

Melt into healing peace now.

'Healing peace' is just another word for
letting go.

**Feeling bad may not have been a
conscious choice, but what about
feeling bad about feeling bad?**
A businessman came to see me and
shared how everything around him
had collapsed. He was financially
bankrupt, his relationship had
broken up, bills and debts flooded
his desk. On top of that, he was an
alcoholic and his health was poor.
As the seconds ticked by, John
recounted his miseries again and
again. It was like a vicious wheel,
everything he thought or shared
revolved around the centre of his
suffering. As he talked, I pointed to
my watch and commented, 'John, no
one could deny you the right to feel
that you are in a bad situation. And
now. . . you were in a bad situation
. . . each moment passing by, you
have a choice how to choose to be . . .
now and *now* . . . and *now*, three
seconds have just passed by . . . how
you choose to be now is your choice!

As he listened, he took some deep
sighs and realized – perhaps for the
first time in his life – that he had this
freedom of choice. He replied, 'I
think I know what you are saying. It
is like compound interest in the
bank. Each moment of negativity can
be compounded.'

I responded, 'You've got it, John. You
could feel bad about having felt bad
and the next moment, you could feel
bad about feeling bad about having
felt bad, about having felt bad . . . Or
you could actually release that old
pattern and start anew this moment
. . . and this moment . . . and this
moment now.'

In this state of release and peaceful
space, John suddenly said, 'I nearly
forgot, I have got a new job offer in
Belfast; I am sure I can still pick up
the pieces and step by step do better.'

There is a John inside everyone,
inside you, who at one time or
another gives up hope and feels
really down. If you are in such a
situation now, gently accept how
you are feeling. You did the best you
could. Your bad feelings of feeling
bad about feeling bad were simply
your way of coping with the
situation and you want the situation
to get better.

Joanne, another T'ai-Chi practitioner,
came out of a shop upset with the
shopkeeper. She was setting herself
up to be upset all day, getting more
and more angry as she walked
towards her car. She decided to use
the Letting Go exercise to release
herself gently from any more self-
criticisms and self-sabotaging
feelings. She was able completely to
release the anger she felt for the
shopkeeper; she realized that he too

Homework 1

was perhaps having a stressful day and that his stress prior to meeting her was unrelated to her. Had she not released these emotions, she might have driven the car in a stressed way and had an accident.

You are an inner gardener with the ability to compost your negative feelings and transform them into your inner garden of peace, health and prosperity

Visualize yourself having a beautiful inner garden; in one corner are your miraculous black compost bins. They will always be here in your heart for you to use any time of the day or night. You simply have to do the Letting Go exercise and imagine yourself letting go any negative feelings you have and placing them gently in this compost bin. Given some time this smelly compost bin will become a smiling bin. At the ripe time, all these ugly substances will be transformed into golden qualities (gardeners call this black gold) to help you grow wonderful, radiant flowers, fruits and vegetables in your inner garden!

T'ai-Chi 'Letting Go' projects can help you attract more peace, joy and prosperity

1 Go into your basement or attic and give away or sell anything you can't use. Letting go of all those things that you do not need any longer makes you feel lighter and more relaxed. You can then open yourself to receive infinite prosperity from the universe.

You need only you to be peaceful. You are simultaneously opening yourself to the Universe (Yin Receptive Principle), to give you useful things which are presently more appropriate to meet your requirements (Yang Emissive Principle). The things you don't need will be freed up to serve someone else. Expect some good, inspiring and enriching situations – projects, relationships, job opportunities – to appear to help you grow more radiant, beautiful and successful. Let the Dance of T'ai-Chi, the dance of Yin and Yang, bring blessings of peace, health and prosperity to your daily life.

2 Start a garden/continue attending to your garden. Respect the Yin Mother Earth energy and prosperity will flow to you. Prepare compost as if it were your inner compost. (If you are unsure about how to make com-post, look in an organic gardening book for ideas.) Through composting you will begin to be aware of how many inner substances can be transformed into valuable

lessons to grow new and exciting opportunities.

3 Practise the Letting Go Exercise every day. Record any insights you have about challenges and inspirations. Note the most serious responsibilities in your life and release them with the out breath when doing the exercise. Your recorded insights may be useful signposts for you or your grand-children to read in the future.

4 For more serious cases of difficulty in letting go, you might like to make a point of seeing two comedy shows a week. If you are at all interested, study the seriously funny art of comedians and understand how they transform hurt into laughter with honesty, vulnerability and love. There are as many different types of comedians as there are of people but, broadly speaking, there is the Yin type of comedian, who loves to be receptive to the audience. And there is the Yang type, who goes through a performance non-stop, unaware of audiences. Many comedians have both Yin and Yang qualities in different degrees.

If you are really daring, try doing stand-up comedy at a local club. If you get heckled and feel like giving up, go back to learning how to make jokes with your own family and friends. It's a good place to practise. Don't get too serious about it. Do it for the fun of it.

☯ *Second T'ai-Chi Exercise/Principle*

Look for balance by accepting your own negatives and positives

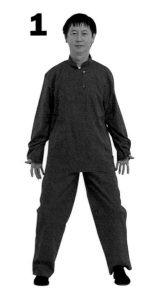

When to practise
This exercise/principle can help you when you feel unsure of yourself and need some wise and balanced decisions.

Best time to practise
Before making important decisions, preferably in the morning or late at night in a quiet environment.

Tao of Indigo Lessons
When you can accept that there are many selves within you that need attention, then you can truly discover selfless service and unity in outward diversity.

1–2 Stand in a relaxed posture. Deliberately and slowly bring your hands behind your back, so that the first finger and thumb touch and form a triangle. Lift your hands up your spine, passing the Gate of Life. This is the place directly opposite

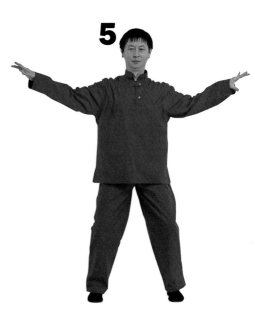

with both arms holding the tension, gradually allow your elbows to sink and turn as you would see a car taking a sharp corner, very slowly.

By sinking your elbows gradually, bring wrists and fingers towards the front. (Optional affirmation: '. . . negatives and all the positives . . .')

2

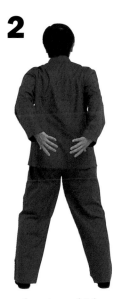

3

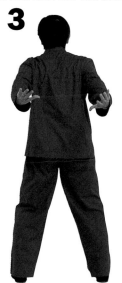

4

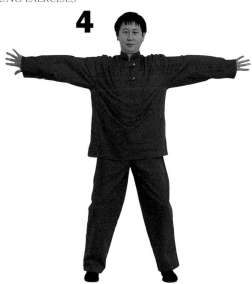

your navel centre, which connects you back to the day you were born into this life. The triangle expresses the unifying relationship between you, your mother and your father during your conception, gestation and birth into this world.

(Optional affirmation: At this point of the exercise, you can say aloud, 'I accept . . .')

3–5 From this triangular formation, gradually release your fingers and

thumbs to connect with the tension of your outstretched arms, like a swimmer about to dive into a pool. (Optional affirmation: Say aloud, '. . . all the . . .') Feel the creative tension of your outstretched arms. Twist your little fingers to point to the sky. Then,

6

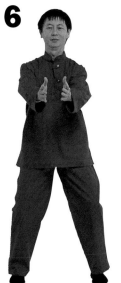

7

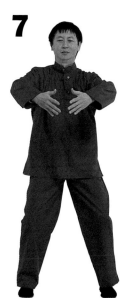

8

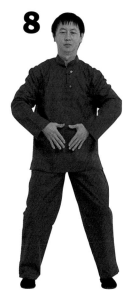

6–8 With your palms and fingers touching lightly (Optional affirmation: '. . . in you, X [speak your own name] . . .'), gently raise your elbows from your sides and watch your fingers come apart

naturally, with the middle fingers still lightly attached, towards your heart. (Optional affirmation: '. . . now!') Pause for a moment and be with your heart. Allow your fingers to slide down very slowly. Why

'slowly'? So that as you glide down from your chest you can thank and appreciate your lungs . . . heart . . . liver . . . spleen . . . digestive system . . . kidneys . . . reproductive organs . . . large intestines.

As your arms fall gently to your sides, slide them to the back again and repeat Steps 1–8. After performing Steps 1–8 twice, go through Steps 1–6 a third time, then proceed with Step 9.

9

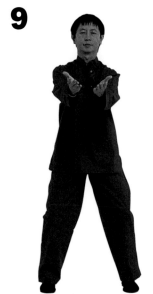

9 Bring your palms to touch each other in front of you as before.

10

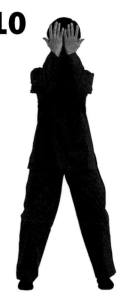

10 Now open your palms in front of your face and hold the two opposite aspects in front of you, as if you were looking into a book with open pages.

14

shoulders, elbows, wrists and fingers are released and composted in the earth.

15

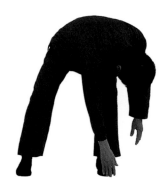

15–17 Bend your knees so that they touch your elbows. Turning from the waist, let your arms and

11

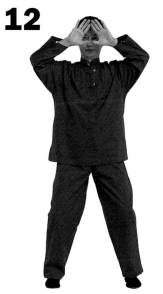

12

13

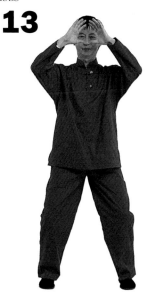

11 Then, close your palms together. In the stillness, feel your peaceful and non-judgmental state.

12–14 From this stillness, open your palms, letting your fingers form a triangle in front of your eyes. Let

the triangle transform itself into a circle, then gradually release your arms so that they fall down towards the earth. The tensions in your

16

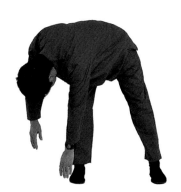

17

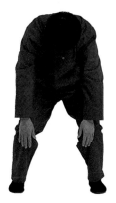

18

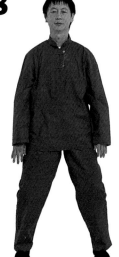

body drop down first to one side, then to the other, then straight down in front of you. Loosen and shake

your shoulders, elbows, wrists and fingers, like leaves falling down from a tree to be composted.

18 Gradually lift up your head and feel your blood pressure returning to normal again.

Hold yourself with gentleness

Can you recall the feeling of wanting to be heard?
Was it the last time when you had a serious problem,
A feeling inside you shouting out, 'Why won't they listen to me?'
They say they do, but you look into their eyes and although you feel their care, you know they can't feel where you really are.

So, who can really understand you?
Where is the solution?
To find the solution to any problem, you need to 'dissolve into a fluid state'.
Water and Air in your body can cross boundaries between enemy camps in your mind,
teach you how to flow with the negative and positive aspects of the situation, and find a third creative unknown possibility.

Please slow down and listen to 'you'?
Where are you now?
Can you feel your breathing and your heart pulsating?
The nature of acceptance is best exemplified in Nature.
Feel how naturally your body does its very best to accept you exactly where you are,
There is already a reservoir of gentleness and courage in your body, accepting all the harmful viruses and bacteria and doing their best to transform the situation into a healthy experience.

When was the last time you held yourself with a gentle reminder of what an incredibly sensitive, intelligent and beautiful world you have within you?

Feel an inner gentleness touching the part of you who is so angry or hurt,
Holding gently,
caring and carrying this part of you.
Feel this gentle touch embrace the hopeful and courageous part of you,
Let these two aspects now gradually melt into fluid oneness.

From this sense of inner acceptance, can you feel an inner space?
So, let a spontaneous solution or idea come to you.
In the mean time, carry on caring about what realistic and practical steps you need to focus on right now.

Why use our names?

Most of us did not have much opportunity to choose our own names. I certainly did not. In fact, I disliked my name. It was too often connected to failure in school or to punishment at home. It was like a special dustbin for all the 'nasties', the smelly stuff of: 'You should be doing this and you should not be doing that, and you could have done it this way and not that way, you *stupid*!' It took me some years of searching within myself, running around in India and the West, to find out that my name was really a wonderful vehicle and not merely a dustbin!

All your life, people have called you by your name: your family, friends, colleagues, strangers who have thought, felt, uttered and read your name in the school register, at the doctor's clinic, from the dentist's filing cabinet and your teachers' report books. All potentially worrying and negative situations. And over the years, your name has been on thousands of envelopes which finally end up in dustbins! Imagine how many hundreds of thousands, if not millions of times, our names and the sound of our names have echoed with all the muddled feelings of ups and downs, pouring more anxiety into them every day.

I first began to realize that a change was happening with my name, when I was studying at the Centre of Personal Transformation at Findhorn, Scotland. When I first went there, I called myself Peter Chin, and the co-founder Peter Caddy introduced me as 'PC of the East'. When I left Findhorn, friends started calling me, 'Choyous One'. Choy is my Chinese name and it used to mean 'Chinese cabbage'! The Findhorn Centre has been known to grow 42 pounds of cabbages, as a demonstration of their love for human co-operation with nature. When I first started transforming in myself, I started affecting other people around me. I cleaned out the old with new feelings of joy and love, transformed a smelly dustbin into a smiley dustbin!

Today, I am still at it. You always have something to clean, rubbish to throw away or recycle. I love it!

Your name is perhaps the most uttered sound in your life and therefore has the most meaning centred round it. Your name is a sound vehicle – actually more important than the most expensive cars, because if you are unhappy with your own name, it is where bad feelings start and can even create accidents. You can choose to accept your name, or change it to something you prefer and begin to use it consciously as a meaningful sound vehicle. You can accept responsibility for keeping your inner vehicle – your name – clean and ready for containing whatever you would like it to contain. You have the power to fill it with creative sounds of gentleness, encouragement, light-heartedness, harmony, self-respect

and peacefulness. These qualities of joy, love, peace, harmony and courage nourish you like healthy food.

Why address yourself by name rather than saying 'I' or 'Myself'?
You are used to hearing your name called, when someone addresses you. You respond immediately, almost mechanically, the moment your name is called. The sound of your name is like a password entering your consciousness and getting you back to yourself faster than any other sound.

Why use someone else's name?
Let us say that you care about someone and that that someone is going through a difficult time, feeling very negative about him or herself and possibly about you, too. One way of bringing about a more balanced situation is to accept that person's negatives and positives from a distance and release the person to be where he or she is. Whenever two or more people are involved in any conflict, this heart exercise helps to bring back an inner balance in everyone concerned. You can do this for a person without them knowing about it. It is as if you were sending a special gift of balance, peace and harmony to a person via an inner airmail system!

Why do the exercise and affirmation at the same time?
The exercises and affirmations come from being in a peaceful, relaxed and happy rhythm. The exercises are

practised from a state of *being* rather than a state of *doing*. In the beginning, people often think that the exercise or affirmation is going to solve a problem, the way a drug temporarily gets rid of the symptoms of a complaint. But I have found that if we ask the right questions, we get the right answers. Ineffective questions create ineffective answers. When a problem arises, do we ask, 'What shall we *do* about this problem?' or 'How shall we *be* with this problem?'

The way we are with ourselves determines what we hope to achieve from the exercise. If we want to be relaxed and, as a first step, we begin to be receptive to relaxing ourselves, then this is reflected in the doing of the exercise. The being principle comes before doing. Isn't this the reason we are called human beings rather than human doers?

Now that we have discovered the importance of being before doing, the next step is to experience the understanding that there is no separation between being and doing. In practising the exercise and the affirmation at the same time, you can speak in a loud and clear voice, or you can say the words internally. Either way, the exercises and affirmations are used to connect the physical body with the emotional, mental and spiritual bodies. Physical relaxation is a reflection of inner relaxation.

Transforming negatives and positives into a T'ai-Chi battery energy

Recently, two people came to see me. They were interested in a private T'ai-Chi class and had some questions. He was a retired technician and his wife a Sunday School teacher. He was 78 years old and she 65 .

I brought out a picture (as in the sketches below) to share with them how T'ai-Chi energy works. Diagram B shows how in a T'ai-Chi generator or battery process, the negative or Yin principle moves towards the positive or Yang principle. In diagram A, the galvanoplastic or electroplating process happens the other way around – the positive 'ions' (the 'I' self is switched 'on') move to galvanize the negative polarity. If you have chrome-plated metal in the kitchen or even gold-plated cups in a trophy showcase, these are produced by the galvanoplastic processes.

He understood immediately, thanks to his background in engineering and electrical work. She wanted to know how this philosophy applied to the T'ai-Chi exercises.

When you shift your weight from one foot to the other, the body weight is gradually emptied from one foot into the other. The heavy foot is Yin/negative and the weightless foot is Yang/positive. The centre of your waist co-ordinates the limb to experience contraction and expansion of energy. You may sense this happening naturally when you breathe in (Yin) – your arms sink and conserve energy. When you breathe out (Yang),

your arms rise up and you feel the energy expanding outwardly. In your emotional and mental awareness, this flow between Yin (negative/heavy/contraction) and Yang (positive/empty/expansion) is the dance of T'ai-Chi.

'Ah yes! A generator!' the technician jumped in. 'You mean T'ai-Chi does what a battery does – generates energy.' His wife asked, 'So, what is this galvanoplastic process? Can you give some examples from daily life?'

I nodded and carried on explaining. 'In the T'ai-Chi Battery principle, you are encouraged to use T'ai-Chi movements and T'ai-Chi principles as pathways into more revitalizing chi energy. A negative problem is accepted with its positive aspect and transformed into creative energy – in other words, a solution to the problem.' I repeated to them to the example of the compost. 'Many people in our classes are also into organic gardening. From the outer garden you can learn to find your inner garden. The outer composting

process of transforming all smelly and negative stuff can be an inner composting process for the gardener.

'In the galvanoplastic process, gold from the golden positive polarity is deposited on the "inferior" metal. The negative/problem is usually solved by someone outside you. Ten years ago, many people depended on their doctors, priests and politicians to fix their problems for them. Today, there are more options, alternatives and variety of solutions available, and people like to try out different ways. But even so, the people who provide the solutions are the golden end of the process. They are regarded as wiser than ordinary people. The ordinary people are the negative polarity. This kind of dependent relationship can easily happen between couples, too. It can also be found in a football game, when the crowd "receives" exciting and powerful feelings of exhilaration from its favourite team when they score. A temporary layer of "golden qualities" of skilful play, light-footedness, harmonious

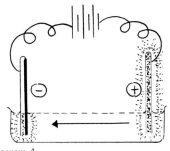

Diagram A
Electroplating battery process

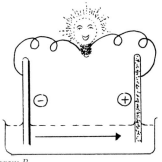

Diagram B
T'ai-chi chi kung battery process

Cigarette smoking and the chi energy experience

co-ordination and heart-centred energy of the players is deposited on the negative receptor.'

The Sunday school teacher added, 'It is true also in religion. People depend on the holy books, godlike presences, images and statues of Masters for the spiritual energy and guidance.'

I carried on, 'Yes, in the galvano-plastic process, the gurus, prophets, high priestesses, kings and queens, scientists and law enforcers are the positive polarity. The disciples and those of lesser knowledge and experience are the negative polarity. In our classes we are aware of these two processes and once the students have learned the exercises and application of the principles sufficiently, they do move on. And they apply this inner generator of chi energy to creative activities in their daily lives – music, art therapy, education, gardening, drawing, decorating etc. We have never created any cult group to keep members under our control. People who study with us go back to their families and apply what they have learned in their existing environ-ment. It is their family members who notice that they have changed for the better – they have become a calmer and healthier person to be around. In fact recently, I received two beautiful drawings from two children thanking me for helping their mum become a more playful and enjoyable person to be with!'

People often associate chi energy with a positive feeling of relaxation, but what happens when you are in a situation when someone is doing something unhealthy, like smoking, and you feel irritated? Can an 'unhealthy' experience like smoking be transformed into a lesson on chi energy?

To illustrate that it is possible to experience chi energy even in such a situation, I would like to share the following conversation, which took place during a T'ai-Chi workshop I gave in France. Half of the group were smokers and the other half not.

Participant: Choy, do you mind if we smoke? I know some people in the group don't like us to smoke. I wonder what you think about smoking and how my T'ai-Chi energy will be affected if I smoke?

Choy: Please may I have your cigarette? Thanks. Light it, please. So, some people have negative feelings about this. And other people have positive feelings about this. Now, I know that cigarette smoking is bad for my health. But I can also sense there is a calming effect that cigarettes have on me. I personally do not smoke, but now, I have this cigarette in between my lips. (I give it a puff . Then I hold it in front of everyone.) So, the question is, can I still feel the T'ai-Chi energy? Let us find out. I have never gone into this question before. I want to find out for myself. Let us see. I need everyone to come closer so that we can find out together. (Everyone gets closer.) Please

come closer. I know not every one of you can, those of you at the back can stand up and come closer.

Look. Perhaps, you can see something happening to my skin, to the hair on the skin. This is an external phenomenon. When you listen to beautiful music, your hair 'stands on end' and you sometimes feel some kind of electrical impulse sweeping (if it is a very inspiring song) into tears of love, don't you?

So, I hold this negative feeling of strong dislike for this object. In fact once I had a dream of it as something I hated, because in the dream someone was smoking a cigarette in front of a baby and I was angry with him. So, now, I hold this cigarette in between my lips – now already a short cigarette, thanks to us looking at it and me speaking so much about it.

I hold this positive feeling about it – it tastes and smells a bit like incense! In my acceptance of both the negative and positive, I breathe in and breathe out, paying attention to the pauses in between the in breath and out breath, OK? Now what happens?

Onlooking participant: Ah yes, I can see your hair on your skin standing like a kind of goose-pimples.

Choy: Ha, ha, ha! Ha! Ha!

Participant: Why do you laugh?

Choy: Never mind why I laugh. The chi

Ah Fook and the railtrack

energy. You felt this same feeling
between you and your musical
instrument earlier, didn't you?
When you were playing your drums,
remember? You felt really inspired and
you felt warm, like a billion tiny little
ants running up and down your spine,
yes? Are we all getting it?

(Long pause . . .)

Choy: Between the sound of water and
the poet or artist, between the rustling
autumn leaves dancing on the road and
your curious eyes. Even between a
feeling of intense dislike and a likeable
feeling? The Tao of chi energy is
everywhere between Yin/negative and
Yang/positive. You have to slow down to
find it. Especially when you need
healing for some pain or suffering, the
inner chi battery circuit within you
needs to connect first.

(A contemplative silence falls over the
group.)

Okay, now, that we are more attentive to
chi energy, shall we do some T'ai-Chi
Chi Kung exercises ?

(The group gets up and we go into
appropriate T'ai-Chi Chi Kung
exercises.)

Once upon a time, there was a little
boy called Ah Fook. His parents
were busy working and had many
children and so Ah Fook went to live
with his grandmother. She
lived about a hundred yards away
from a disused railway track. Many
people used the railway as a crossing
place . Children loved to hop on the
tracks in the evenings after school
and invent jumping and racing
games. Ah Fook was also lucky
because right in front of his granny's
place was a big playground. He was
just one year old and beginning to
walk and talk. Each morning his
grandmother would take him to the
playground and watch over him.

One day, while Granny was talking
with the neighbours who had also
brought young ones to the playground, Ah Fook walked to the old
railway and sat down to play. He
was pleased because he did not fall
down even once. Ah Fook seemed so
happy and contented sitting there.
Passers-by could hear him making
chuckling sounds to himself.

The postman, who knew the family
well, came by and said, 'Ah Fook,
what are you doing here all by
yourself? Your granny will be
worried.' Ah Fook's smiling face
looked up; he was pointing with his
little finger at something in front of
him, but the postman walked away
to the playground to let Granny
know of Ah Fook's whereabouts.

A student late for school crossed the
rail and looked at Ah Fook. He

exclaimed, 'Lucky you, you don't
have to go to school,' and then he
skipped off.

Soon, along came a familiar figure.
And Granny too. She stomped over
to the railway and was about to
scold Ah Fook for being naughty
when she saw a man who had
stopped nearby to see what the little
boy was looking at. Granny knew
this man well: his name was Wang
and he travelled widely and bought
precious jewels and clothes from the
East to resell them in the West.

Wang beckoned to Granny to
observe the little boy. Ah Fook
looked up with beaming eyes and
pointed gleefully to show Granny
and Wang what he had found. He
was looking intently at the polished
rail track. Granny was puzzled and
wondered what it was that had
intrigued the little boy intrigued.

Wang explained: 'Look carefully, do
you not see the little specks shining
like jewels on the polished track. Ah
Fook is in bliss because he can let go
of any previous perceptions about
the railtrack. He can feel the lightness and the brilliance of those tiny
specks on the iron surface with
his whole being. It is as if he has
become one with all the stars in the
universe.'

Granny smiled as she took the little
boy's hand and asked the wise man,
'Would you like to walk back with us
to the house and have some food?'
Wang nodded his head approvingly.

Homework 2

1 Draw a line down the middle of a sheet of A4 paper and write down a list of negatives and positives about how you feel. It could be about a difficulty you are experiencing in a relationship – with a partner or ex-partner, or with your parents – or something to do with your work. This helps to bring a balanced awareness of your Yin and Yang polarities *on the feeling level*. Initially it may be difficult to think of the positive aspects of this exercise. You may need to go for a walk and take some time off before coming back to your piece of paper to reflect on what positive lessons you have learned from the relationship. Write as much as you need to, depending on how much negative feeling you have.

2 In front of a mirror, sketch ten negative and ten positive aspects of yourself. This helps to build an awareness of your Yin and Yang polarities *on the visual level*. If after some attempts you feel you cannot draw very well, slow down. Take another look at the main features on your face. Notice perhaps your hair, nose, ears or lips – any parts which seem prominent – and draw those in first. You need only ten minutes to half an hour for this exercise the first time. Then leave it and come back to it after a day or two.

3 Laugh with yourself in front of a mirror. Make faces at yourself – an angry face, a happy face, a peaceful face, a sad face, a supportive and loving smile, a childlike grin, a stern look, a mad look, etc. – and have a good laugh. When was the last time you laughed at your own dualistic nature?

4 Before any undertaking that makes you nervous – such as speaking to a group of people or going to meet someone important – write down or mentally refer to the opposing 'push and pull' aspects within you. Use the Second Fundamental T'ai-Chi exercise mentally or physically to accept your own negative and positive aspects before you embark on whatever it is. You can also do this reflective exercise after the event to help you learn to be more confident next time.

☯ *Third T'ai-Chi Exercise/Principle*

How to let go of self-criticism and accept yourself as you really are

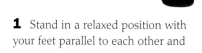

1

When to practise
This exercise/principle is a very gentle way to get back to a feminine, nurturing and accepting attitude.

Best time to practise
In the midst of your work schedule or travelling in a bus or train, you may find the section of this exercise where you place one palm on your physical heart beat and the other palm on your lower abdomen very comforting.

Tao of Blue Lessons
Let the qualities of peace and clarity bring you closer to your real self which is truly non-judgmental.

1 Stand in a relaxed position with your feet parallel to each other and about a shoulder-width apart. Sink down until your knees are over your toes.

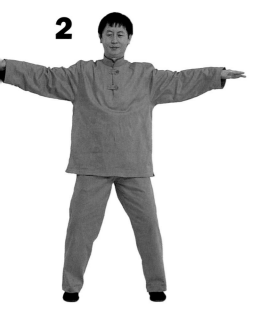

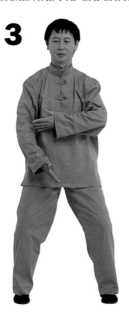

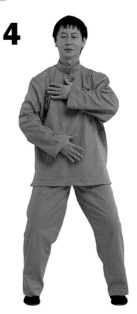

2 Allow your elbows to open up and raise your lower arms, like a bird opening her wings.

3–4 With palms facing down, gently bring your hands back to tuck the right hand just below the left elbow.

Your left hand should be about 7.5 cm (3 in) from your chest. Lift your arms up again as in Step 2.

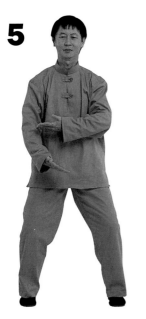

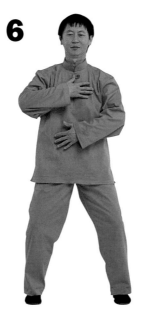

5 As you sink your knees down, lift your arms again as in Step 2.

6 As you let your arms fall again, sink your knees by another 2.5 cm (1 in). Reverse the position of your hands, so

that your right hand is on your chest and your left hand on your stomach. Now go through Steps 1–4 again. When your arms fall, sink your knees a further 2.5 cm (1 in). Then repeat the whole exercise three more times. This time, when your arms fall, raise your knees 2.5 cm (1 in) further each time. On the third repeat, your knees will be back in their original position.

Promoting a non-judgmental attitude and state of being in Wu-Chi (emptiness)/Tao (fullness) 'I love you and I accept you as you are'

The fourth exercise with the principle, 'I am love, you are love, all is love' (see page 53) can be used in conjunction with this principle.

This non-judgmental accepting attitude can work only when you apply it firstly to yourself. I realize now that for a long time I really didn't understand what a non-judgmental attitude meant. I was constantly surrounded by reminders of self-blame in school or at home, and of blaming others in the news on the radio, television and in the newspapers. Whenever there was any crime or problem, there was always a search for the culprit – who is to be blamed for this?

I recall a vivid example of a time when I was making a small bonfire in my back garden. My neighbour leaned over the wall and shouted at me, 'Why are you making that fire, all the smoke is going in my eyes!' I had heard myself talk like this before, and I recognized the blaming tone of voice. It has echoes in people from all walks of life and cultural backgrounds. We all know it so well. It is around you like a gloomy cloud because you have got it *inside you*!

The challenge for me was to accept my neighbour as he was and to feel my own sense of not knowing what best to do (the Wu-Chi empty feel-

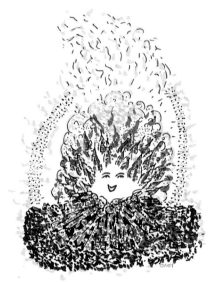

Fire chi energy
Fire chi can either burn us and others with blame and bring clouds of gloom and doom or it can be used wisely to bring nurturing warmth, forgiveness and compassion. The choice is yours.

ing). So I asked him sincerely about how the smoke and fire disturbed him. He said that he had just come home from work and after a hard day's work, he wanted to relax. Then, this smoke came into his face.

I accepted that this was unpleasant for him, but I also knew that we had checked with the local authorities and they had said we could make a fire as long as it was not too big and that we lit it after 4 p.m. And this is what we did.

I told my neighbour that I really wanted us to win together in finding a solution which would suit both of us. So, I offered to make any fire later in the evening when it was too cold for people to sit outside. By approaching the problem from a non-judgmental point of view, we had seen a third possibility which was acceptable to us both and this gave us a feeling of satisfaction (the fullness of the Tao Principle).

This succeeded because I had worked on my blaming selves first (even though my neighbour might not have). Whether my neighbour liked it or not, I was going to do my best to get us what we both wanted. He was genuinely contented with the solution. Somehow it got through to him that I sincerely wanted us both to win.

The T'ai-Chi art of walking
What was it like to walk with the ancient Taoists? What would it be like to feel your every footstep a tingling joyous experience? You feel privileged to walk silently besides the Masters. Everything has a dream-like quality; your feet feel as if they are gliding on the road.

I used to wonder why my teacher U G Krishnamurti was called a Tai-Chi Master even though he taught no special traditional T'ai-Chi Chi

Kung exercises. The only exercises we did were walking, cooking, sitting down – all normal, day-to-day activities.

Let me tell you how I met him. I was at Putthuparti, India, in the ashram of Sathya Sai Baba. One night I had a dream and in the dream, I met a man walking along a road towards me. I said hello. He nodded a greeting. I felt there was something very wise about this man. I turned to face the direction he was walking and walked beside him. We walked together for a short while. We spoke softly and gently. I remember wishing that I could see his eyes. I thought to myself, 'I know, I am going to invite him to have a cup of tea with me, and I will sit opposite him.' I asked him. He nodded in agreement. There was a little tea place in front of me. As I sat opposite him, I eagerly looked at his eyes. Suddenly, I felt myself soaring out into the universe. I felt an

indescribably exhilarating sensation of being one with billions of stars. And I heard myself scream out, 'M . . . A . . . S . . . T . . . E . . . R!'

When I woke up the following morning, I met someone who shared with me about U G and told me I must go and see him. I was given an address. When I finally met U G up in the mountains near Bombay, he came to greet me and take me to his lodge. While walking back with him back, I suddenly stopped and exclaimed, 'But . . . but you're the one I met in my dream!' I told him the dream and he simply nodded without speaking. We carried on walking silently up the road – just like in the dream.

I lived with U G and three other people – a lady called Valentine, an American and a German man. We had visits from people who came to U G for healing and for advice. During one of our walks, I was

astounded to notice that the 'head part' of my shadow had disappeared and only a white glowing shape remained where the head was supposed to be. I played a peek-a-boo game with this phenomenon by going into the shadows of trees to see what would happen. My head remained white even under the tall trees! And the glowing white space was also there when I came out into the sun. The rest of my body had a shadow, but not my head!

I have asked other T'ai-Chi and Chi Kung Masters in China about this phenomenon. It is known in Chi Kung practice as a very advanced stage of development. Although today my head shadow has returned to the rest of my body, I do still occasionally experience the white space, as if just to remind me that that state is still there. This phenomenon is about the head being willing to let go and return into a Wu-Chi state of nothingness.

Learning to listen to your heartbeat can bring more health, peace, love and joy into your life

I started learning heartbeat listening when I met U G. Before I met him, he had undergone a physical transformation which defies logic. Some of my Taoist Chi Kung Masters in China explained that when the chi energy reaches a point of saturation within the physical body, a total transformation occurs on a physical, cellular level. Doctors in Switzerland had pronounced U G clinically dead, but three days later

they discovered that he was alive. They examined him in a medical laboratory and found that his skin became literally luminous. They also found that his internal organs were in excellent health.

People experience different results from learning this simple heartbeat-listening exercise. One person heard music in her heart. We pay so much money to book or join long queues to

buy opera tickets to hear some famous soprano or tenor sing. Would opera lovers pay the same amount of money to hear their own hearts sing? Another student of mine who did a lot of heartbeat listening, thanks to a machine he was hooked on to in hospital, could hear oceans, seas and rivers splashing and flowing. He was literally shaken up by the experience. He exclaimed, 'there is so much bloody flowing energy inside me!'

We were never taught that we could actually hear, feel and *be* in our heart organ and hear music or feel warmth and have *fun*! In schools, colleges, universities, clinics and families we are given the limited view that the heart is just another physical part of ourselves. As you grow older, your heart could prove to be a unique lifetime friend. Many of us have not been educated to love the heart we have until it is a little too late.

Not long ago I heard a report on some recent medical research which indicated that one out of three people in England would die of a heart attack. Apparently, someone in England suffers a heart attack every three minutes! The researchers attributed this to too much cholesterol, the result of a poor diet. Not surprisingly, in a country where lots of people eat deep-fried fish and chips on a regular basis.

However, when they compared the statistics with Japan, where people consume even more cholesterol than the British, they were surprised to find that the Japanese have a lower heart-attack and heart-failure problem. The big difference is that the Japanese believe in working eight days a week, while the British need their tea breaks and are always striking for better pay!

These statistics suggest that the solution lies not so much in improving our diet but in the correction of physical inactivity by doing more regular exercise. However, there is surely more to this problem than meets the eye. Let us think about the question of 'putting your heart' into what you do.

When people are not motivated, feel anxious and uncertain about their future, they naturally 'lose heart' and are more likely to fall ill. Successful people who work hard may be burning up calories and cholesterol, but surely it is more important for them to feel motivated in their job, to be able to say, 'I love my job wholeheartedly.' It is only natural that you should love eating wholesome food cooked by happy and heartfelt cooks. My father had a restaurant and he taught me that it was always important to get to know the cooks if you eat in a restaurant. So, I am happy to share with you that there are many wonderful, happy and loveable cooks out there. Could you be one of them?

If you have balance, radiant health and vitality inside you, you can only express that in the way you cook and in the balanced recipes and ingredients you find in order to prepare your meals. And, naturally, you look for that sort of quality cooking when you go out to eat. Have you ever seen a balanced, happy meal coming out of a stressed-out and sour-looking cook? Of course not. One look at him or her and you have lost your appetite!

So, the practice of heartbeat listening can bring you closer to your heart and perhaps motivate you to do what you really want to do with your life. And enjoy it. You will also be able to practise it in relation to finding the right kind of healthy and balanced diet you need. Heartbeat listening can help you decide how you cook, what you want to cook and which restaurant to choose next time you go out to eat!

Taking heart-felt steps in your life

Imagine a day when whatever you do, you do it from an inner sense of harmony and peace. You have made the decision to feel caring and with your whole being you have decided to look for the best things in life to appreciate.

Each second that passes, two million new mature red blood cells enter your circulation to maintain normal blood supply in your whole body. Isn't that an amazing thing to give thanks for? When you step on the pavement ready to go to work, every cubic millimetre of your footstep has more than five million red blood cells totally supporting you. Even though you may not be aware of it, your heart is pumping blood at 75 beats per minute, carrying precious nourishment to the whole body and helping to get rid of wastes. What a miraculous organ the heart is!

From your heart, feel your chi energy flow within your blood, carrying billions of messages of appreciation to every cell.

Feel this in your arms, your hands, your neck, your legs.

Feel harmony in the way your feet are moving.

Feel peace in the way your heart pulsates.

Feel chi energy throughout your whole body.

All through your life, your parents' lives, you as a child and as a parent will always receive an abundance of harmony and peace in your body. Even when you are unwell, your body does its very best to keep on caring. In your heart, you know this to be true.

Heartbeat listening livens up boring meetings and dull functions

Have you ever counted the number of meetings you have gone to, which are so boring and so dull that you wished you had not gone? If you wrote them out, you would not be alone in having a pretty long list. There are also the dull functions and parties which everyone else seems to be enjoying, but are they? How often have you felt that superficial atmosphere in the air when someone greets you with a polite 'How *are* you?' You have no desire to answer because you know that the person really doesn't care how you are. Well, I don't know about you, but I have certainly felt this.

Do business meetings *have* to be boring? Can the heart transform serious topics on the agenda into interesting discussions?

I have served as member, secretary, chairman and president of many committees, groups and societies, and I believe that it is possible to put the heart into meetings. When we tried this, meetings really did become more productive and interesting. Okay, you say, what about boring items like minutes? Well, there are practical steps that can be taken here. Items on the agenda which do not require in-depth discussion could be posted to participants beforehand. Minutes

of the previous meeting can then be read at your own convenience. When people meet, there is so much between them that goes unspoken. What keeps people focused and enables them to achieve communal goals is, I believe, the underlying warmth, fellowship, laughter, affection and the fact that they share a heart-felt purpose.

So how do we create this kind of heart-centred atmosphere? What happens when the members of the group decide to close their eyes and listen to their heartbeats for a minute before starting the meeting? Is that not a logical way to start if you want people to put their hearts into whatever they are supposed to do? If they do this, the quality of heartfelt energy will naturally flow into the products and services connected to decisions made at the meeting.

At the end of the meeting, you can also make a heart-to-heart pulse connection by holding hands for a minute or so. This will enable everyone to feel the heart meridian connecting with everyone in the group before saying goodbye. This simple group exercise can help to create a core of heart energy in the group. Each person stretches out their left hand, palm up, to receive the chi warmth from the person on their left. The right hand faces downwards, sharing warm chi with the person on the right. And then, you can reverse it. This encourages a supportive and circulating stream of chi energy among the individuals in a group. The Yin (receiving), Yang (giving) and Tao (creative) chi energies are activated to help the group succeed in whatever they want to achieve.

When the chi energies flow from left to right – anti-clockwise – they are concentrated and strengthen the purpose of the group. When the energies flow in a clockwise direction, they expand the chi outwardly and energize the creative actions of the individual group members.

How do you know if chi energy is flowing in the group? Chi is felt as an electrical kind of current of energy passing through your palms and fingers. Most people start off by feeling some tingling warmth in their fingertips. You can also feel more chi flowing when the palms and fingers are barely touching each other.

Heartbeat listening can help heal stress

She was in her sixties. She walked with hesitating footsteps, her eyes half-blind and half-closed. She also had sunglasses on. She was slowly dragging her steps up the staircase to the therapy room.

She started sharing. 'My mother is in her eighties and I go every day to help her. She is half-blind. I developed similar symptoms of semi-blindness when I started going regularly to see her.'

I joked, 'I know someone who loved monkeys a lot and cared for them in a very devoted and loving way. People also noticed this person walking and looking more and more like a monkey after some years!' She laughed.

She complained of pain in her eyes. Lying down on the couch, she placed her palm on her chest and started listening to her heartbeats. I placed my palm on her hand. Together we listened to the throbbing pain in her eyes. It was as if the eyes were telling us a story. As she breathed in deeper and deeper, with this gentle awareness of a tender warmth pulsating from her heart, the pain left her. I put my palms over her eyes and heart region. I could feel a gentle healing radiance over her whole body.

An hour later, she opened her eyes and shared, 'I feel a lot of light. Thank you. Thank you for the healing. I feel no more pain in my eyes.' When she walked down the stairs, her footsteps were firm and steady. She did not need her sunglasses as she walked out into the delightful sunshine.

Two days later, she phoned to say how healed and peaceful she felt. She had slept soundly for the first time in many years. When she went to see her mother, some of the pain in her eyes came back again, but it left her as soon as she went home. She took one of my tapes on heartbeat listening and told me that it had helped her to take rejuvenating and peaceful naps.

The heart has an immense capacity to teach us how to rejuvenate and how to flow in loving energy. Scientists know that your blood makes one complete circuit of your body every minute, travelling through 60,000 miles of veins and arteries! A small area like your eyeball contains over a million intelligent little beings called cells, being born, dying, with new ones born again by the millions; they were working day and night to keep this lady alive, so that she could experience meaningfulness in her life. What splendour of colour and life eyes bring into our lives! So much to be grateful for. As gratitude increases, chi increases through the blood. Chi

repairs, rejuvenates and activates healthy new cells.

Heartbeat listening can help set you free – and let your heart sing!

Jay, a performer, used to be afraid of crowds. Thanks to heartbeat listening and the Second T'ai-Chi Exercise of accepting the negative and positive, he started enjoying the audience and the audience enjoyed his performances. How does it work?

Listening to the pauses between our heartbeats allows us to rediscover open spaces in our consciousness. These inner spaces allow us to feel free. All artists, musicians and creative people seek this inner sense of freedom in order to create. It extends outside and makes people like Jay feel free to sing with all their heart. In fact, it is as though your heart is doing all the singing, and therefore the voice feels effortless. Jay went on to learn how to connect his heart energy with his breathing from his belly centre, to experience an even more effortless flow of harmony in his performances. He became a heart-throb to many of his fans! If you have not discovered the singer in you, heartbeat listening may be able to help you.

How heartbeat listening can help you in times of danger

When I first started learning T'ai-Chi, my daily energy discoveries taught me the home truths of the T'ai-Chi principles. One night I was walking home at about 9 p.m. The side streets were lined by corridors between the shop fronts and the market stalls on both sides. The vendors had packed up their stalls. As I turned into one of these quiet streets, a harsh voice called out from

the shadows, 'Hey, you, come here!' I stopped in my tracks. My heart was pounding like an African drum. I did not know what to do, except to listen to my heart. At first, I could feel waves of panic going through my body. Then I listened to the pauses between my heartbeats. This calmed me down. The voice called three more times, getting louder each time.

I did not move. Listening to the pauses between my heartbeats brought a deeper and deeper feeling of peace to my whole body. I also felt no more fear. It was as if paying attention to the pauses 'paused' the consciousness. This really puzzled the guy who was shouting at me. Why was I not moving, not reacting to him at all?

Finally, he came out from the darkness and angrily demanded why I did not go to him. He also asked if I had any money to give him. No response from me again! By now, he was infuriated. His head edged closer and closer to mine as he insisted on knowing why I was not answering him. By this time, his voice had a slight tinge of nervousness as he stood there puzzled over my silence. Up till then, our eyes had not met. When that maximum point of curiosity was reached, I gradually lifted my head up and our eyes met – eyeball to eyeball. No words. No sound for a few seconds. It was as if time stood still. I felt no aggression or fear in my eyes. His eyes looked confused and afraid. A few more seconds of silence. Then it was all over. The silence had won. I patted him on the shoulder and said calmly, 'Next time, watch who you shout at. Good night.'

The yielding/receptive T'ai-Chi energy and houseflies, birds and mosquitoes

I am by the river Ganges, Benares, India. How did I get here? I have been visiting the wisemen of India, the Yogis. After practising my T'ai-Chi and Chi Kung, I sit down. There are millions of houseflies. I keep very still and watch these little buzzing insects investigating my face.

I am watching my reaction to them. I have been brought up to believe that houseflies are 'bad' because they carry bacteria and spread diseases. These reactions bubble up inside me like lava from a volcano. My fear of the insects has to do less with concern about harmful bacteria than with the irritation. This itchiness! And flies seem to love eyes! I stay very still and watch my impulse to want to chase them away. One part of me, the Yang aspect, wants to swipe at the flies and make them leave me alone! Another part, the Yin aspect, wants to be loving, kind and peaceful with them. This stillness, and my awareness of my dualistic response brings a flow of chi energy. I can feel it all over my face. It enables me to transcend the irritation. I wonder how the flies are taking all this buzzing chi energy all over my face, eyes and body. It seems to have calmed them, too. After a short while, they leave me without my doing anything to them.

Another day, I am sitting by a large tree, in a quiet, Yin/receptive state. I am not concentrating on any particular subject. Suddenly, I feel a bird's voice singing in my heart. I feel my heart is bursting with song, beauty, joy, harmony and love – all at the same moment! All this happened in a matter of ten seconds and then it was over. The bird on the tree flew off. I felt dazed and dumbfounded. The awareness of oneness was spontaneous and effortless. There was no preparation, no visualization and no special technique. When the mind and emotion are in an effortless and naturally quiet Yin state, the outside world is experienced as 'not separate'. The outside world, which is normally in a Yang state, is suddenly discovered to be at one with the Yin state. There was never any separation in the first place.

I have had other similar experiences. Once when I was walking in my home town, Kuala Lumpur in Malaysia, I noticed some workmen digging a ditch on the other side of the road, just outside the bus terminal. Suddenly, a wave of terrible sadness came into my heart and I felt the pain of one of the workmen. He was an elderly man trying to use a heavy pick to dig the ground. I felt tremendous compassion for him.

Another time, in Scotland, I passed a puddle on the road after the rain. I suddenly felt a beaming light smiling in my heart.

Whether they seem positive or negative, I feel that all these experiences are like new seeds being sown in my heart's inner garden.

As the years went by, I began to discover that I could *choose* to have these experiences, rather than them happening to me spontaneously and without warning. I learned to use a minimum amount of 'light effort' to achieve what I want in my life. Let me give you another example. Back in Malaysia, we had houses on stone and wooden legs. When I was a teenager, I found a secret place for meditation – under the house. The only problem was that it was not a secret from the mosquitoes!

The mosquitoes used to land all over me. I noticed my instinctive reaction: 'I'm afraid of these little vampires!' I accepted this part of me who wanted to swat at them and slap them. But there was another, opposite part who wanted to make peace with them. I chanted very softly, 'You are peace, I am peace, all is peace.' I accepted these two opposite parts of me and went deeper into a contemplative stillness. I started to feel chi energy pulsating through my whole body. Amazingly, the mosquitoes stopped buzzing around me. The chi energy seemed to affect them! Might they be meditating too? Or were they asking themselves, 'Hey, what's up with this? Why doesn't he or his body fight us? And what is this strange energy pulsating through us?'

In our science class I recall setting up the anode and cathode (positive and negative) polarities of a battery and connecting them to the bulb. I see this as an appropriate analogy to explain how T'ai-Chi works. If you embrace the negative and positive inside you, you will be able to feel the chi energy flow and then, when there is sufficient flow of chi energy, you may feel your head light up like an electric bulb! You will naturally and effortlessly feel more energized, harmonious and at peace with your environment. And you may find you know how to deal with people in your daily life who are as irritating as mosquitoes!

Allowing the yielding/receptive T'ai-Chi principle to protect you

When I started learning T'ai-Chi, like many teenage boys, I was interested in martial arts. After only a few years, I was doubtful about how the T'ai-Chi yielding principle could apply in a real-life situation. And then, one day while I was walking in the crowded streets of Kuala Lumpur, a guy came up behind me and grabbed me, demanding money. I did not have time to think. All I saw and felt were my two hands spontaneously repulsing the attacker from my back; he fell on the road-side. Someone else came towards me from the front and also attempted to grab me; he found himself flying off my body. All this happened in a matter of seconds! It was not at all like in the movies, where you see and hear the kicks, punches and defence moves in slow motion with exaggerated screams and tomato juice flowing as a substitute for blood. Only when the two people I had fended off got up and ran away did I realize consciously that I had been attacked!

I found myself calling out to them, 'Hey . . . you!' I was amazed, to say the least. And probably they were too! They ran into the crowd. Later, upon reflection, I realized this experience explained what Professor Cheng Man-Ching, Grand Master of T'ai-Chi Chuan, said, '. . . some T'ai-Chi exponents have what is called the Receptive Energy, the attacker is repulsed spontaneously.' It was as though an attacking force had boomeranged back into the attacker, not through any conscious act of mine but in an instinctive way.

A real street-fighting situation can happen so fast that the conscious mind cannot keep up with the action itself until it is all over. In some cases, knowledge of fighting techniques may give one a false sense of confidence. The T'ai-Chi art of learning to accept the *unknown* force and learning to flow with the aggressive force is totally different from other martial arts, which emphasize preparation by rehearsing possible *known* directions from which the blows and punches are coming – you learn to condition yourself to tackle them with blocks, counter punches and tackles.

The T'ai-Chi exponent is like the painter who paints in an unknown state of consciousness and is surprised when the painting draws a lot of unsolicited appreciation. Like the painter, the T'ai-Chi artist looks at the masterpiece with genuine surprise: 'Did I do that?' In those moments, the absence of the 'I' from the past allows an intelligent and appropriate response. In the absence of the self-conscious 'I', the artist can melt into the moment and produce something absolutely fresh, new and inspirational. In contrast, if the artist only imitates past painters, he or she feels second-hand, third-hand, and is recognized only for doing good imitations. In a first-hand experience,

the T'ai-Chi exponent looks at his hands, feet and body as an unknown feeling of energy pulsating through his whole being. Ancient T'ai-Chi Chi Kung Masters state that this unknown chi force is intelligent, fresh and alive. To keep continuous contact with this force, you have to let go of your past and be in the ever fresh, new and unknown moment-to-moment way of living. You need to learn to trust it to protect you, to nourish you and to energize you whenever you need energy.

This unknown force operates within clear laws of Yin and Yang, as are stated in all Chinese medical texts and philosophy. What is not explained clearly is why it seems to be so mysterious. No matter how great an artist is, the painting of the sunset can convey only a very slight impression of the grandeur of the real sunset, which was disappearing as the artist painted it and will never be repeated again. T'ai-Chi is truly an ever-fresh and new art of living and being one with chi energy.

Around the same time, to give another example of my relationship with chi energy, I was working as an assistant librarian in a secondary school. It was my first job. Besides a lot of filing and library duties, I enjoyed reading in the reference library section. One day, when I had finished my work, I remember locking up the library on the second floor and walking downstairs. Then I heard some Lower Sixth Form girls calling for help. They were surrounded by a group of older secondary school boys, who were taunting them. I went to them and asked them to stop. They did. And they turned their unwanted attention on me instead. Some of them stood in front of me and jeered at me. Another group went behind me. One of them gave me a hard push on my back. The moment I felt the push, my right palm went up in slow motion and turned very slowly with my body to face the attacker. I felt as if my right palm was carrying a ton of bricks! All the boys seemed to feel it and one of them shouted out, 'Look! Look at his hand! Let's run for it!' And they did.

Although I felt the power in my hand, I did not expect them to react in such a dramatic way. This incident showed me once again that aggressive forces can be absorbed, concentrated and boomeranged back. One interesting addition to this experience, is that the rhythm of my response was very slow, whereas when I was attacked on the street it was very fast. In fact, in this incident, my slow movement felt to me more powerful than the fast movement. Once again the sudden appearance of chi energy surprised me.

Homework 3

Morning or night meditation for 15 minutes

1 Practise the first three fundamental T'ai-Chi exercises for about 10 minutes every day.

2 Describe the Third Fundamental T'ai-chi Principle in your own words. How are the Yin, Yang and Tao principles connected to this third principle?

3 Begin today to affirm that your natural immune system and natural sympathetic nervous system are doing their best to help you heal any ill condition in your body. When you wake up in the morning or when you are at home in the evening, send to any part of your body that feels ill or stressed the message, 'I love you and I accept you as you are.' You and everyone around you (including doctors, nurses, friends and relatives) will be doing their best to help you.

4 Bring your palms up to hold your heart and belly centre. You can do this exercise lying down or sitting up, and use either hand. Pay attention to the pauses in between your heart beats, and to your in breath and out breath.

5 Spend a few minutes acknow-ledging the presence of the Wu-Chi within you. If you feel the sense of aloneness or loneliness within you, embrace it with peace and stillness.

6 Observe any thoughts and feelings that come up in you. Use a mirror to look at the different selves coming up. You may see a tired self, a worried self, an insecure self, a hurt self, an angry self, a frightened self. Affirm verbally, 'I love you and accept you as you are.' Behind these selves is the need for loving acceptance. You are affirming what you already are. You are a happy, loving and accepting self.

Space to record your own insights

☯ *Fourth T'ai-Chi Exercise/Principle*

Learn the art of receiving and giving with love

When to practise
When you sincerely want a loving answer to conclude a situation with someone you care about.

Best time to practise
In the evening when you feel mellow and inward.

Tao of Green Lessons
Allow Mother Nature to embrace you in loving, harmonious energy.

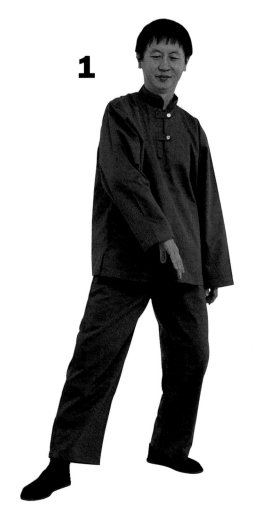

1

1 Standing in a relaxed posture, with your heels together and toes pointing out in a V-shape, allow your body to sink into your feet. Take a step forward with your right foot, leaving your left foot where it was.

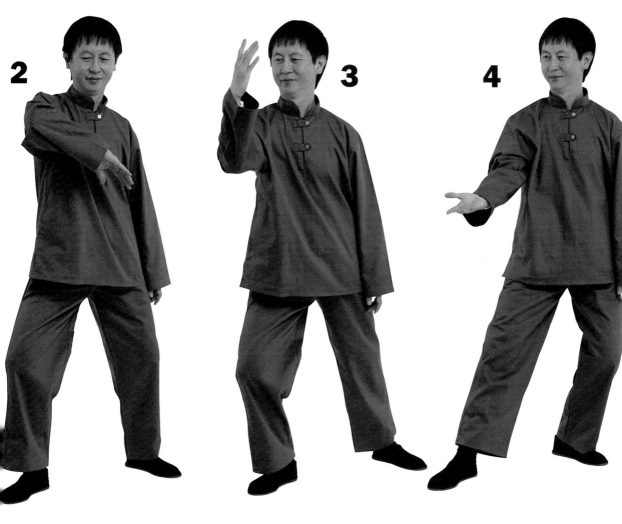

2 Transfer all your weight into your left foot. Turn your right hand, thumb and first finger to touch your tan-tien or navel centre.

3 Slowly, draw up your right hand from your elbow. Turn your elbow upward, as if it was being pulled from above. Move forward, turning your waist slowly to the right at the same time. Allow your elbow to fall gently and slowly. As it sinks, allow your wrist and palm to follow. Feel your fingers open up. Your palm is opening

as if you are offering a flower. The weight of your palm is supported by your elbow. Feel your palm and fingers tingling. Feel the gentleness of the wind. Your fingers may feel as if they are touching velvet, as they glide through the air. The air is filled with trillions of atomic particles of vibrating energy. Scientists tell you that this is a fact. You are a bundle of energy, but do you feel it? Do we give ourselves the time and space to discover this fact, first-hand?

4 Gently guide your palm down. Let it fall lightly, like a leaf floating down in slow motion. Feel the gentleness of the wind or air supporting your arm. Turn your waist inwards, shifting your weight back to your left foot. You are know in the same position as in Step 1. Repeat the exercise, using your left hand and left foot, and facing towards the left.

The Fourth Dimensional Experience

It is as if you have a garden there inside,
starting from the roots in your feet up
your legs,
Tan-tien flowing wheels of energy,
Chakra mandalas of radiant flowers on
your palm,

Your whole body is in your hand.
It feels like the most exquisite musical
instrument ever created in the universe.
What a gift, what a joy it is to move,
every gesture is a unique musical
masterpiece no sound in thought or word
can capture.

The rhythm of touching your belly, heart
and mind
gently throws you into an electrical
shower,
waves of delightful smiles welling up
from within you,
melting you into tears.
They are here, you feel them,
radiant presences of uncountable ones,
luminous, secretive and free they dance
around you.
Where do they come from?
The passing breeze through the window
sending shivers up and down your spine,

your palm rising up like a hurricane in
slow motion.
Ever slowly, like water vapour rising
and falling raindrops,
your hand dances down, down, like
leaves even slower down to the earth.

Hot warm tears rolling down your
cheeks,
the feeling of pure, gentle love all
around you,
the unearthly smile spreading across
your face from the inside out.
You are amongst friends of light.

The tingling T'ai-Chi hand
Chi energy allows you to feel that your
whole body is tingling in your hand.

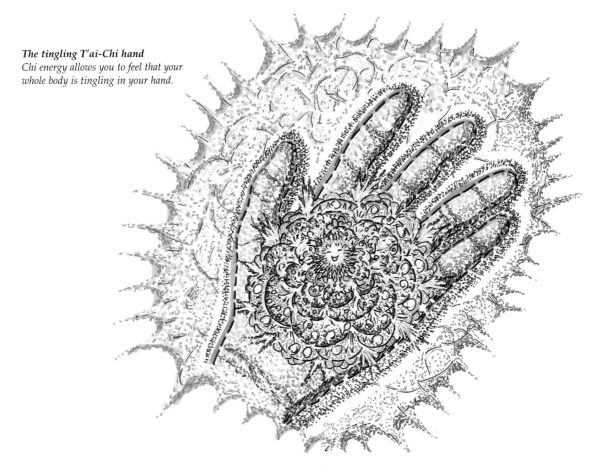

The four dimensions and stages of evolution of yourself

The first dimension is where you see only one point of view, whether or not the point is positive or negative. It is still only one dimension. In a symbolic sense, it is like looking through a rolled-up poster.

The second dimension is when you can begin to sense 'two sides of a coin' in every issue. All political, economic, educational, social and scientific views keep alternating between right and wrong, good and bad. One party or person seems to be wrong while the other believes they are right. One group feels satisfied and happy with the deal while the other side feels badly treated. One group seems to overwhelm the other. The challenge is to move from a state of domination and submission to learning how to flow with each other. Ultimately this becomes like a dance.

In the third dimension, you feel more in balance. Now, you are able to see three sides to a question. There is a

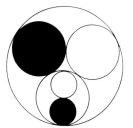

The dance of Yin/ Yang into T'ai-Chi and Wu Chi

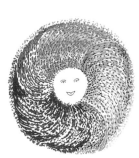

Being Number 4 – the true chi energy self

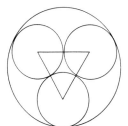

Equal-sided triangle, a synthesis of the Yin/mother, Yang/ father and Tao/child principles

third synthesized possibility to every issue or problem. There is a flow, a dance of Yin and Yang, the negative and positive transforming into a dance of receptivity and action. T'ai-chi shares the same flow of Yin and Yang as other kinds of dance in many cultures. The difference is that T'ai-chi places more emphasis on the slowness and fluidity of the movements. This dimension is also about the awareness of the unknown. In Chinese, it is called the Wu-Chi, the

Great Void. From it comes the freshness and spontaneity of relationships.

In the fourth dimension, you get to the centre of these three sides, like finding the centre of an equal-sided triangle. That's the Being Number 4. Say 'Hello' to him/her inside you! It is like going home to find your parents and your childhood self waiting. 'Welcome home,' you hear them say. Hugs, kisses, warmth, lightness and laughter. All one.

How the 'I am love, you are love, all is love' principle was discovered

In 1978, I had a dream of being chased by negative feelings. These feelings were like a wild wind running after me. I recall, in this dream, that I was running and running and running and then, suddenly, a voice stopped me in my tracks and said, 'I am love, you are love, all is love.'

I felt my whole being pulled into this wheel of sound, which kept on chanting the same words again and again until it turned into a wheel of love and light. All the negative feelings that had been chasing me disappeared. Ever since then, I have realized the tremendous practical value of this sound.

I have used it in business, in social life, in stress management, in my relationships with the people closest to me and in application to whatever happens around me. Over the years this sound has made such a difference in my life that I could not envisage any day passing without using it. So, how does it work?

In the beginning, it was like a gift from the Almighty and I was never quite sure how I should take it. It was too simple, it seemed to drive home the importance of linking up 'I' and 'You'. These two polarities of 'I' and 'You' exist for most of us. Our thinking and daily inner conversations are filled with thoughts and feelings of about what other people ('You') think of us ('I'). The constant chattering mind, I found, was chattering from a standpoint based on the separation of 'You' and 'I'. What do You think of Me? Am I good enough for You? Do I satisfy You/Your expectations? What do You want from Me? What can I get out of You? All these questions occupy our inner agendas in daily conversations with friends, relatives and strangers, whether it is for socializing or for business purposes.

So, this sound, 'I am love, you are love, all is love' first of all unifies and brings together the polarities 'I' and 'You' with the 'All'. Does this mean that you are God or something? No, you are not separated into a God as opposed to someone else who is not. A river cannot be contained in one cup. You can swim in the river and feel a sense of oneness with the river, but only the river can be truly the river.

The next stage of my understanding of this sound was seeing it as a tool that I could use, for example, when I faced a formidable client. I am thinking of a certain man who was reputed to have cheated my company; he did not want to pay his debts and was as nasty a person as you are ever likely to meet. My boss challenged me that no one had been able to collect the money this particular client owed. I used the tool of 'I am love, you are love, all is love' and, with the help of colour science, collected the dues.

Fluke shot? Well, they sent me again and again and every time it worked. I helped that company, which was

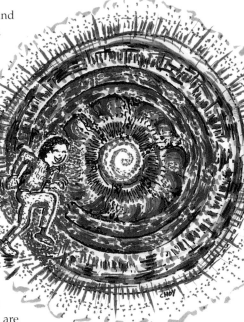

Entering the fourth dimension of oneness and love

down in the dumps because of all the debts, to become a 10-million-dollar business with award-winning trophies alongside their financial achievements. And I was working for them as an account executive, not a debt collector.

But although I was handling a large number of clients and promotion was imminent, I realized that my true vocation lay in sharing this tool and my interest in T'ai-Chi. I was already teaching people in business and my friends how to find more relaxing ways to live their lives.

How to use the 'I am love, you are love, all is love' in business
Before a meeting begins, for example, visualize a light connecting you with the person you are going to meet. (The light visualization is the Yin/feminine principle; the sound is the Yang/masculine principle and the creative principle is the harmony.) Chant 'I am love, you are love, all is love' in your heart and in his/her heart and allow the loving concern between you to guide both of you to a caring and co-operative business dealing. It is even more effective if you have learned the colour science of drawing the qualities and colours you want to see manifested in that situation (see page 144). There is always care behind the handling of a client, a product and the team of people who are going to help you accomplish what you want to see happening.

How to use the 'I am love, you are love, all is love' when driving
Safety belts and expensive insurance policies can help you in many ways when you have an accident, but do you not think that ways to prevent accidents are equally important? The collective fear of motorists will sooner or later find a vehicle to express itself. Fear and worry are used like preventive tools to get us to avoid accidents. You worry in order to express your concern.

Concern?

Yes. Basically isn't concern one degree or a deeper degree of expression of love? You can decide for yourself which is more effective – using a negative to get to a positive result or using a positive to get to a positive result? So, you can visualize a positive, light-hearted feeling at the place you are driving to or in the people you are going to meet at that place. Chant 'I am love, you are love, all is love' silently to yourself for a minute. Connect the light at the place with the light in your heart and the car with the light of the sun. This also creates a reassuring feeling between you and your car. Loving, protective energy links you up with your destination and helps you to arrive safely.

How to use the 'I am Love, You are Love, All is Love' when you leave your children at home with a nanny or babysitter

When you realize deep within, that you do have a choice between fear/worry and loving concern, and the two do not need to mix together, you can trust in the power of the loving energy to be there taking care of your children at home when you go out. You know that you have done your very best to ensure that anyone staying to take care of your child has a caring and loving attitude. By chanting 'I am love, you are love, all is love' in your heart when you leave your loved ones and connecting the chanting energy with the person taking care of them, you affirm that the loving energy is protecting them. Of course, this chanting does not in any way take away our right to feel naturally anxious or afraid, but our anxiety or fear becomes like a catalyst to help us learn to be wiser and more prudent in our ways of taking care of our loved ones.

The story of Light Beam

Once upon a time there was a beam of light, called Light Beam, that came down to the earth from the Heavenly Light. It was lost and looking for a way home. It was not only feeling lost, it also needed to connect with other brother and sister light beams.

Light Beam saw a beautiful diamond deep in the earth and jumped into it and felt how beautiful it was. But after a while, Light Beam realized it was not really home.

Then, it saw a dewdrop on a blade of grass and thought, 'How lovely!' Light Beam danced into the sparkling dewdrop and felt its transparency and purity. After a while, Light Beam realized that this too was not home.

And then, Light Beam saw a child sitting on the grass, crying and crying. Big teardrops fell down from her cheeks. Light Beam flew into her tears and felt all her loneliness, all her feelings of loss and abandonment. Light Beam cried with her and felt all the love of all mothers for her. After a while, Light Beam realized that this too was not home.

Just then, the parents of the child arrived and shouts of jubilation were heard and tears of gladness shed. Light Beam went into the tears of the parents and thought, 'Yes, yes, this must be home!' Light Beam felt the happiness of the parents and the child reuniting. But after a while, Light Beam realized that this too was not really home.

The parents had asked a clown to come and entertain the child and her friends to celebrate the lost child being found. The clown was painted with bright luminous paints and had colourful jewellery on his clothes. Light Beam thought, 'Oh goody, surely this must be home!' It raced into the clown's luminous paints and shiny jewellery and felt the freedom, joy and lightness. But after a while Light Beam realized that this too was not really home.

So it came out of the clown and looked up at the universe and said with all its being, 'Please, please, won't you help me to find my true home?'

A great silence followed. Then, suddenly Light Beam felt itself glowing brighter, bolder and lighter. It was like a droplet of water realizing what it was like to be the ocean.

Light Beam became a little star. The more it knew that it had the feeling of being at home within itself, the more it shone. And it became so bright and cheerful that it filled everything with joy and felt a sense of oneness with every other light beam shining in everything on the earth.

Why is it difficult to experience oneness?

Many people I have met share how they experience an ecstatic feeling of oneness with Nature when they go deep into their meditative movements in T'ai-Chi Chi Kung. They feel a physical sensation of oneness with trees, animals and the universe. Some even describe how they gave up their dependency on alcohol, coffee, cigarettes or drugs without any effort. Many people also share that they feel envious of this first group of people and ask, 'But why doesn't it happen to me?' Let us use T'ai-Chi principles as a mirror to know ourselves better.

First of all, let us examine this fear of surrendering, letting yourself go totally into the meditation. You have the fear of surrendering into someone else's control. People experience the swing between fear and faith when they think about surrendering to a master, to a god, to a saint or whatever, but this is not the kind of letting go which we are talking about. The fact is that unless you have learned to trust yourself to surrender to the courageous and loving energy within you, there will always be the fear of surrendering to some outer or higher force. A T'ai-Chi student of mine (who is also a dedicated Christian) shared recently with me that she felt Christians often forget the last part of the verse in the Bible which says, 'Love your neighbour as you love yourself.' This is based on the assumption that you are loving yourself. But are you? Do you? What does it feel like really to let go, to love yourself and trust your gut feeling? Once you can do that, you become an initiate rather than a follower. Another student shared about how he helped an old man quite spontaneously and later felt as if he were helping part of himself. An initiate is someone who initiates creative projects and ideas, who makes inspirational activities happen. The more you learn to trust your gut feelings, the more you open yourself to trust the universe and receive harmonious guidance.

Then, you move into the second dimension of holding the polarities in your life. It is as if you are learning to use your legs all over again. You have emotional legs, mental legs and spiritual legs. You learn to hold the negatives and positives in your life, and balance yourself to find solutions to conflicting situations. In other words, you grow up from being a baby to become a child who can start to walk, to eat, to rest, to play and to communicate. You can see yourself as an emotional child, a mental child and a spiritual child. An emotional baby merely cries when he or she is hurt or hungry or feels lonely. Having grown into an emotional child, you start to learn to heal your hurt with love and feed yourself with appreciation and self-worth. A mental baby is one who depends on others to feed him or her with intellectual stimulation.

The mental child learns to think for him or herself and comes up with imaginative and new insights to old problems. A spiritual baby is praying for a saviour and looks to the coming of the Chosen One. There is a longing for a mystical union with the Master or with God. A spiritual child begins to know his or her own innocence and plays with light, love and joy in the world.

In the third dimension, the creative spark is accepted as the norm. Many diverse paths open to the initiate and he or she learns to love and accept his or her own limitations of time and place. In this stage, he or she is learning the value of patience and persistence. There are many kinds of fruit trees, shrubs and vegetables to take care of. The initiate accepts the value of ripe timing and opportunity for the growth of every project and seed idea. There is also a need to link up with other people, to help each other to grow and share plenitude and inspiration on the emotional, mental and spiritual levels. The child grows to be a teenager. The emotional teenager learns to support and co-operate in order to achieve what he or she wants. The mental teenager not only comes up with bright ideas but is willing to sustain those ideas and commits him or herself to starting and completing the projects. The spiritual teenager is an enthusiast, an adventurer who accepts the unknown as a source of inspiration. Initially, there is a rebellious attitude, but this is a temporary state of restlessness. The initiate transforms the unquenchable and thirsty type of relationship into something creative and interactive.

In the fourth dimension, the artist, the brush, the paints, the canvas and the scenery become one. The emotional teenager, now grown into a young adult, is like the artist who shapes and moulds reality into an eternal, loving, orgasmic celebration. The mental young adult is like the gardener who lovingly tends and supports the heart to collect new seed ideas and grow their unique blend of lovely qualities with Nature.

The spiritual young adult stands tall, strong and radiating loving inspiration for those around him or her, as a beacon lights the way for lost ships and boats.

Homework 4

1 Practise the first four Fundamental T'ai-Chi exercises every day for at least 15 minutes. Describe the First, Second, Third and Fourth T'ai-Chi principles in your own words.

2 Give three examples from your daily life as to how you have used the first three T'ai-Chi principles.

3 Explain how the first three T'ai-Chi principles connect to the fourth principle.

4 Practise chanting 'I am love, you are love, all is love' for about 10 minutes every day or whenever you feel you need to.

5 Write down an example per week to illustrate how you have used the Fourth Fundamental Principle to make yourself more effective in achieving what you want.

6 Write down any instances when you have used these tools to help someone in a stressful situation.

Space to record your own insights

_____

_____

_____

_____

_____

_____

_____

☯ *Fifth T'ai Chi Exercise/Principle*
Use the effortless way to achieve what you want

When to practise:
This exercise/principle is useful when you feel unclear about your goals or feel too attached to what you want to achieve and need to let go, relax and simply be your self.

Best time to practise:
In the evening when you come back from work or whenever you need it.

Tao of Yellow Lessons:
May wisdom guide you upon the path of humility.

1

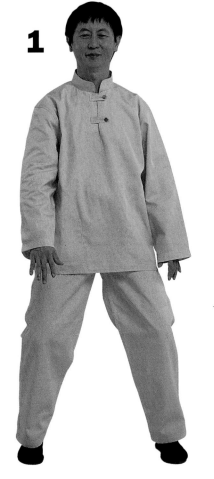

2

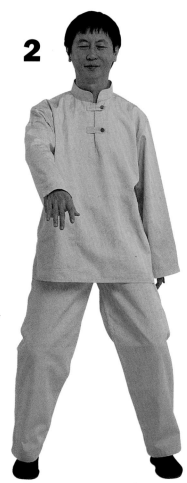

1 Stand in a relaxed posture with your feet shoulder-width apart. Swing your arms gently by your sides, as if you were going for a walk.

2–3 Moving from your waist, throw your arms up in slow motion, one arm at a time. Your aim is to throw your hand up to touch an imaginary point right in front of you. Keep practising this throw from the centre of your waist. Allow your first finger to touch that imaginary point.

4 Continue until you succeed in making it such a smooth movement that it feels like a seagull gliding on a sea breeze, as your hand glides down in slow motion. This exercise will help your improve your concentration. Nothing escapes your eye when it is focused on the path of

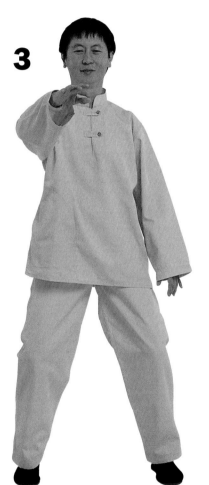

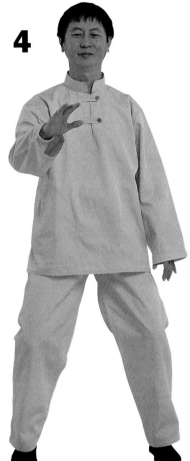

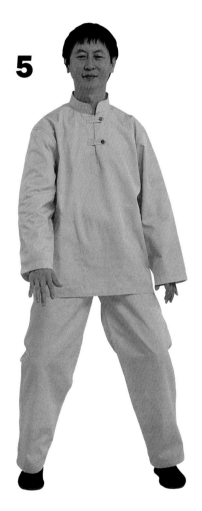

your swinging palm. Your hand feels every minute sensation – no matter how clumsy or beautiful, it is recorded in your awareness. As you drop your hand in slow motion, you realize that you have touched and released your imaginary goal.

5 Now you can allow your hand to return to the side of your body. You do not need to hold on to that which you desire most. You can release it, as if you were lovingly releasing a beautiful caged bird so that it can sing and fly freely and naturally and

fulfil its fullest potential. You touch the happiness of freeing your inner birds, your most cherished goals and noblest ambitions. An arrow cannot find its target until it is released from the bow.

'I touch my goals and release them now'

One person's goals may be very different from another's. One may want to find an ideal partner. A man who is divorced may want a second chance to start a new family and be able to support his previous family too. A woman who has lost custody of her daughter to a jealous ex-husband may want to rebuild her life and work towards the day when her daughter will come back. Another person may want to be reunited with someone who has passed away. Yet another may simply have the goal of passing an examination or finding the right job.

Someone who is in debt may be concerned only with prosperity and abundance. And even if some people have the same goals, they each feel differently and have uniquely different hopes about that goal.

Achieving the goal of self-healing

Linda had been medically examined by doctors with the latest technology and found, to her horror, that they had accidentally severed one of the main nerves in her hand. Her fingers were paralysed and she lost her job. Linda's goal was to heal herself. Together, we saw how remarkably she released herself to touch and realize her goal. She saw that her goal was not to complain about what a terrible mess she was in. She wanted to release all the feelings of blame.

The chi healing hand
Every physical cell in our bodies is made up of an infinite number of chi energy particles. Chi energy is intelligently reorganizing, repairing, transforming and helping to accelerate the healing.

Linda went through the first dimension and principle of learning how to let go of her role play of blame and inner hurts (see page 28). She worked on the second dimension of accepting the negative and positive aspects of the whole situation. She accepted her inability to go to work for the time being. She did her best to get compensation from the doctor and hospital who had put her into that situation. But she also discovered that she could transform this useless arm into an excellent opportunity to learn about self-healing.

Together with other complementary therapists, we did the best we could to help her help herself. Each week, we encouraged each finger to move with chi energy. We shared the joy of seeing not only one finger moving – at the end of about five weeks, the hand got back its colour and all the fingers could move and grasp. Linda had realized the goal of the healing, of joy, patience and persistence.

She did not give up hope. When she went home, she practised and practised holding and letting go of a glass. She was learning how to touch and release her goal just as her lifeless fingers were learning how to hold and let go the glass to exercise her finger muscles.

There are infinite ways of going all out to get what we want. Linda put her whole heart, body, mind and spirit into achieving what she wanted and she got it.

The Dance of Light in your eyes

You may discover that on some days your mind cannot stop chattering. Chatter, chatter, chatter. Worry, worry and worry. Anger. Your lips vibrate with words. Your voice may not correspond with your thoughts and feelings. What people say may not be what they mean. Fearful eyes mislead. Unsettled eyes awake from nightmarish dreams. The inner light becomes vague; unclear feelings of loss, anxiety and panic can overwhelm us. How do you return to the inner light in your eyes?

Firstly, let us find out which comes first, sound or the light of vision. The T'ai-Chi principle reminds us that light is the first step of consciousness in action. Sound follows pictures. Pictures are made from light and colours. How do we bring back this natural balance, to put light first?

A simple step is to practise *verbal fasting*. A silent day. Speak less and less. Speak only when absolutely necessary. Use a notebook to write down what you want to say.

This silence works like a movie projector projecting light, colour and sounds on the screen in your mind. Reduce the volume of the sound level more and more, and you will begin to notice more and more the light rays between the screen and the movie projector. You can adjust the intensity and clarity of the quality of picture on the screen. This is what a verbal fast can do. Gradually, you notice a greater respect for silence and the subtle world of light and pictures.

There are different intensities of light. You can find the intensity which suits you best. It does not matter whether the inner pictures feel good or bad. They come from the light and energy source. Return your eyes to the world of pure light and energy. Outwardly, you may begin to take more notice of people's eyes.

The Dance of Light in your eyes is beautiful. You forget what a person looks like, what dress she is wearing, you forget her hairstyle or her age, or the job or problem that she has. The Dance of Light in your eyes is so simple. It is too easy for us to take our eyes for granted and forget the biological fact that *eyes love light*! If you are with someone who would like to try this out, right now, turn to that person and notice this inner light of beauty in his or her eyes. Be in silent appreciation and see if you can feel the way his or her eyes love light.

Emotionally, also, many young people are hungry for attention. Attention-seeking behaviour can be either negative or positive. Recently, a schoolboy convicted of stabbing and killing a headmaster was discovered to be someone who loved to create trouble just to attract attention. Young people seek the light of attention – and sometimes they go over the limit. Performing daredevil acts or committing a crime becomes a means to attain more thrills and admiration from friends and foes. On a socially more acceptable level, fashionable clothes and flashing disco lights hold out the promise of a good time.

As you grow older, your ambitions may turn towards winning golden cups and awards, passing exams, promotion at work, a respectable position in school, college, university, church, office, a new house, new furniture, etc. And this stirs up the look of awe, envy and admiration in all. The light of approval from the eyes of the peer group is something to strive hard for. Otherwise, you can get heavy looks coming at you, like heavily laden dark and shadowy clouds hiding the sunlight of hope and fun.

There is nothing wrong with aiming for all those wonderful light-filled things. The challenge is when we forget that the light of approval comes from the inner light. I only want to bring you back to your eyeballs and have a ball doing it! Go to your eyeballs and notice this amazing inner light of love dancing when you think about someone you admire with all your heart. Do you feel the inner light dancing between you and the one you admire? Look inside now, can you feel this inner light glowing in your heart? Feel it. Let it glow for its own sake. Let it glow in your eyes, on your face. You are gradually becoming conscious of a picture of light behind all pictures of your loved one.

Relax into the inner light. Realize that you are a dancer of light in your eyes. No matter what your thoughts and feelings are, let them all melt back into this source of light. You are a beaming source of light energy. Enjoy this peaceful radiance. Nothing to do. Just be in this glowing light.

Homework 5

1 Practise the first five Fundamental T'ai-Chi exercises for at least 20 minutes every day.

2 Explain in your own words what is the galvanoplastic process. Give five personal examples of how the galvanoplastic process has occurred in your daily life.

3 Pick out instances in the field of entertainment where the entertainers have successfully used the electro-plating process.

4 In your own words, what is the T'ai-Chi battery process?

5 Give five personal examples of how you have put the T'ai-Chi battery process into practice.

6 List three creative projects that make your heart sing and jump for joy! Write down clearly the steps you would take to achieve them.

a One project should connect to your Yin aspect, to help you to increase your feminine and intuitive sensitivity. It could be doing a painting class, taking up music, writing, T'ai-chi, yoga, etc.

b Another project must connect to your Yang aspect, to empower your masculine side. Do something to serve other people in whatever capacity you can. This could be a family project – renovating your house, decorating the bathroom, etc. Or it can be part of a larger community or global project.
c The third project must connect to your creative Tao aspect. This could take the form of something which makes you enjoy your creativity in a dynamic way – playing, dancing, singing, getting married or whatever.

7 Keep a journal and write down your progress through the projects. Describe the development of your Yin, Yang and Tao aspects within each project.

8 Also record how long it is going to take. A reasonable amount of time for three serious projects could be nine months. Some projects will obviously take less time, while others take longer to mature. You could make a week-by-week plan of what you will be doing for the next 36 weeks.

Space to record your own insights

☯ *Sixth T'ai-Chi Exercise/Principle*

Release your old perceptions and allow yourself to be as you really are

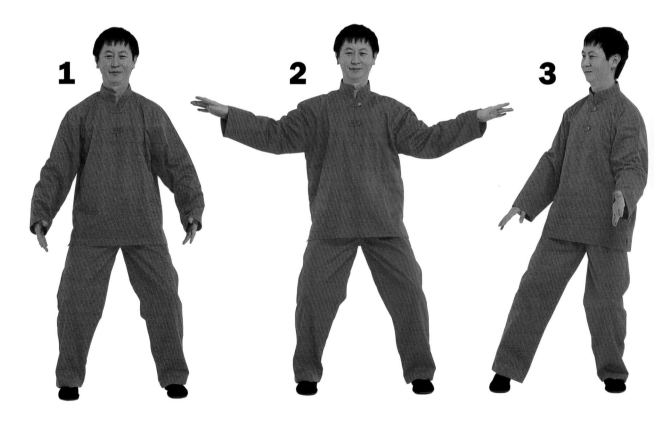

1 **2** **3**

1–2 Stand with your feet about shoulder-width apart and swing your arms around your waist. From the centre of your belly, with a gentle flick from your waist, lift your hands to your sides

3–4 Slowly drop your hands down, like a leaf falling down in slow motion. Turn from the waist and face towards your left.

When to practise:
This exercise/principle is applicable in situations where you or someone you care about needs emotional space.

Best time to practise:
In the evening, when you come back from work, or whenever you need it.

Tao of Orange lessons:
Melt into happiness right now. The path home is happiness. The space around you is happiness.

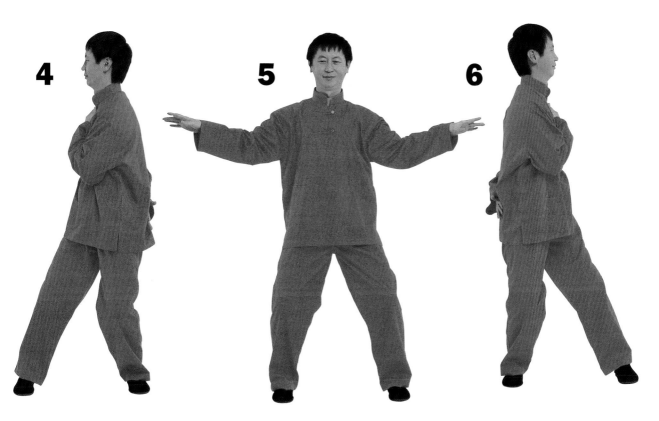

5–6 Turn to face forward again and allow your arms to open up like an eagle in flight. Then allow your hands to drop down again to your sides.

Start again. Do your best to keep both feet parallel and rooted, especially when you turn your waist.

How to use the 'I release you to be as you are now' principle

You have gone through the first dimension of looking at life from a one-biased perspective into a second dimensional way of perception. This means that you are capable of seeing two perspectives. Then you experience the centre of that triangular viewpoint to get a fourth dimensional experience of life. From here, you can use the energy to touch the fifth dimension, which is about touching your dreams, your goals of wanting to be more loving and happy. Now, you have reached the sixth dimension, where you release this beautiful new qualitative energy of loving and joyous fulfilment to be embraced in your heart and body.

A meditation to help you create a space for yourself to be

After reading this passage, you may like to close your eyes and feel inside. How do you feel right now? Whatever you feel is OK. Feel it as it is. If it is an anxious you, a fearful you, a guilty you or an uncertain you, just be there with these selves as they are. They are like children who have been longing for acknowledgement.

The more you are aware of your responses to outer events, the clearer your inner landscapes will be. Feelings of blame are created by a 'blaming self'. This blaming self seeks acknowledgement and release from its negative state. When you hear yourself saying, 'I am worried and I blame myself/him/her,' what you really mean is, 'I am concerned.' There is genuine concern behind the worry. The self is by nature loving. When the release is given, when the inner self behind the worry and blame hears you saying to it in a sincere tone, 'I release you, X [your name], to be as you are. I love you as you are. You do not need to change for me to be caring,' you give this inner self the right, the permission to be as he or she is, to be accepted as loving. Then sit back in the stillness and watch what happens inside.

Take a pause and feel what this means right now.

Using 'I release you to be as you are now' with your partner

We all know whom we love in life, but sometimes we forget to release the people we love to be as they are. How many parents would love their children to be successful and happy, but forget that what their children really want from them is the freedom to pursue their own dreams and to realize them in their own ripe time? And when you as the child grow up to be a teenager and adult, you may discover yourself having the same attitude towards yourself. You have not learned how to release your creative self to be as he or she is.

You can use this exercise focussing on someone you love. For example, if you love Mary, you could say, 'I release you, Mary, to be as you are.' This could be the best Christmas and birthday present you ever gave her! This is a feeling. Do not go home and tell your loved one, 'Right, I am releasing you. I am going to pack my bags and leave!' When you release that person to be as he or she is, the person will feel it and relax better with you. So, if you would like to, close your eyes now, visualize your partner and affirm, 'I release you, [his or her name], to be as you are.'

If you use this affirmation and principle, your loved one will not feel pressured and strung up by your expectations and hopes. The silence between you will be easy and gentle.

'But I don't have enough space to do all this. There are so many problems and pressures around me!'

If you are going through a crisis, you may feel that everyone around you is pressurizing you to make decisions and this makes you feel you do not have enough space. When you look more closely into this lack of emotional space, you will see that you have loads of it. You have plenty of emotional space – the problem is that this space is often taken up by worries. Lift up your arms and let go of the worries. Go within your consciousness and let go of the urge to find fault with the person(s) involved. What you get as a result is lots of creative space.

This exercise also has a lot of benefits for people who want to have a wonderful digestive system. A lot of feelings of negativity are stored in the stomach region. Taoists believe that fear in the kidneys, anger in the liver, worry in the spleen and nervousness in the intestines can be neutralized with chi energy.

When your arms come down, brush across your belly centre, let your chi energy flow through your belly and spine. It will help to improve also your appetite.

The Dance of Perpetual Motion

When you really release yourself to be as you are, what happens? You discover for yourself that you are made of tingling energy. Scientists agree that everything, including your body, is a constant perpetual motion of atoms, molecules, electrons, protons, neutrons, quarks and so on. In a word – energy!

Whatever you do, whether it is learning a T'ai-Chi exercise or performing any other movement, no two gestures of your body are ever the same. When you try to memorize the movement, you get an approximate idea of what it is and then you keep repeating it. You crystallize your understanding of it and in doing so you burden yourself with expectations. You may feel frustrated in the beginning. You think that the problem is that you have forgotten what you are supposed to be doing. But in fact you are experiencing T'ai-Chi as a Dance of Perpetual Motion.

If there comes a time when you have practised this dance for ten years or more and you suddenly think and feel that you really know the movements, then at that moment you have stopped learning. Remember that life is in a state of perpetual motion.

Nothing stays static except what we hold as our memories. What you *are* can only be discovered when you let go of yourself. People practising the T'ai-Chi form sometimes forget how to practise being in the T'ai-Chi formless essence. The first step is the last step. The Dance of Perpetual Motion is happening even when you are not doing anything to do with T'ai-Chi.

Often when we get stuck on some problem we find ourselves feeling heavy and bogged down. No matter how hard we try to get out of the situation, we end up feeling even more stuck. Once we learn to release

this sense of 'being stuck', we find we can produce a solution. It may be something we have never thought of before, and yet it suddenly appears so simple and relevant. This kind of honest gut feeling comes when we learn that it is okay to let go and let the Dance of Life sweep us off our feet into a new step!

Let your whole life change simply because it is changing. Let your face change. Let your fingers, toes, ankles, calves, thighs, hips, abdomen and chest change. The universe is forever young, beautiful, intelligent and secure. We can join or not join this dance whenever we want to at any given moment.

Right now, you can simply let go, let go of all that tightness in you and let energy and a sense of lightness come into your awareness. Realize that this is how your body really is. Melt into it . . . consciously, let yourself melt into this ceaseless, moving

Homework 6

energy, which is not something that you imagined, but is really happening right now.

Can you feel it? Can you feel your face changing? Move your head and neck in a gentle spiral manner. Feel that your spine is soft and pliable. All your blood cells are in a Dance of Perpetual Motion. The moment you let yourself go into it, you will feel.

Take a breath . . . pause . . . take another breath . . . pause . . . take another breath . . . pause . . . take an even gentler breath. Feel your breath to be a ceaseless dance of energy. Feel your belly breathing. Let your breath dance in you. Let your arms and hands move with this breath.

Now, let go of all attempts to move. Just be, simply be with an awareness that your face is changing . . . relaxing . . . and trust that change is the way of Nature and the way of the universe.

If your body feels like rocking gently from side to side, let it. It is unnatural to make your body keep still. Relax and gently spiral your body with your belly centre like the centre of a buoy floating in the sea of life. With your feet rooted to the ground, rejoice quietly in this expansive space. It is you. Sink into it. Melt deeper into it. Breathe it. Use your breathing like a ladle to scoop up some chi energy and quench your inner thirst. Or just lie back and relax into it. When you feel it buzzing all over you, it will feel like a jacu-chi bath   and that is better than any jacuzzi experience.

This cosmic chi energy is not something to be serious about. Have fun with it. Move into it and out of it. Once you have tasted it, you will never lose it again, because is as if it is recorded in your taste-buds. It is like the best home-cooked food! You can celebrate it with a toast to the Cosmic Comical Cook. Cheers!

1 Practise the first six Fundamental T'ai-Chi exercises for at least 30 minutes every day. Write down any insights.

2 Describe in your own words what the Sixth Fundamental T'ai-Chi Principle is.

3 In front of a mirror, light a candle and focus on accepting the inner Light Being inside you. Let this inner Light Being be released to be as he/she is. Let your eyes, lips and whole face light up into a smile. Affirm verbally, 'I release you to be as you are.' Do this once a day in the morning or evening.

4 Write down five people whom you would find it difficult to let themselves be as they are. Towards the end of your daily 30 minutes' exercise, when you are doing the Sixth Fundamental Exercise, verbally affirm, 'I release you, X, to be as you are', inserting the name of each of these people.

Space to record your own insights

_____

_____

_____

_____

_____

_____

_____

_____

_____

_____

_____

_____

_____

_____

_____

☯ Seventh T'ai-Chi Exercise/Principle

Create your self-esteem with sincere appreciation

When to practise
Whenever you feel depressed and you want to see golden lining on the grey clouds.

Best time to practise
In the evening in conjunction with the other exercises, especially before doing the eighth exercise.

Tao of Red lessons
Be courageous with every loving step you take in life. All the colours of the rainbow radiate in you beautifully right now.

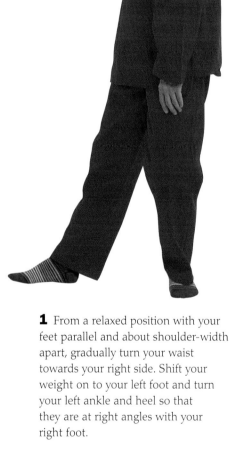

1 From a relaxed position with your feet parallel and about shoulder-width apart, gradually turn your waist towards your right side. Shift your weight on to your left foot and turn your left ankle and heel so that they are at right angles with your right foot.

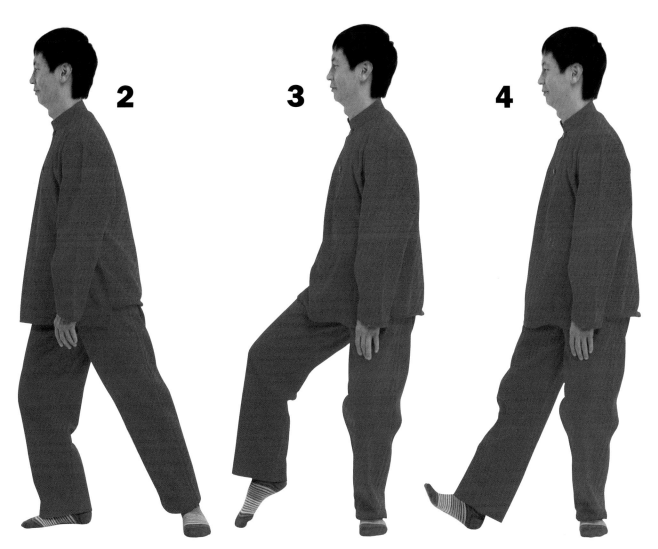

2 Without lifting your foot, gently shift your weight on to your right foot. Keep your soles resting flat on the ground. Now slowly and gently shift all the weight of your body from your right foot back to your left foot again. Keep your shoulders square and your eyes looking straight ahead. Pause, then shift your weight back to your left foot, then back again to the right. Do this seven times.

3–4 Now, keeping all your weight on your left foot, lift up your right foot so that it is resting on the toes, then pivot the foot back so that it rests on the heel. Do this combined toe-to-heel movement seven times.

Turn your waist to the left, shifting your weight to your right foot, and repeat the exercise on the other side.

Seventh principle/dimension: the thanking process

When I was growing up, my father and other relatives would often share with me the importance of being grateful to Nature. When we went into the jungle to collect medicinal herbs, we would thank the Nature spirits in the plants. My father also brought home wise men who meditated in the jungle and they too advocated this attitude. Being grateful and giving respect to the mountains, rivers, rocks, insects and all life is not restricted to the ancient T'ai-Chi Chi Kung philosophy. It is also taught in other ancient traditions – among the Celts, the Druids, Native Americans and the Aborigines of Australia, for example.

Human beings have the ability not only to receive but also to give appreciation. The more you give, the more there is to receive and finally it boomerangs back to you. The balance of giving (Yang) and receiving (Yin) is an effortless universal principle working to your benefit when you begin to use it.

Appreciate what you already have
Take a pause and recollect everything you have. You may be surprised how many things you can think of. Start by being aware of your body itself. What do you have? Your limbs, your internal organs, count them one by one. Listen to your heartbeats and your breathing.

Appreciate the simple things you have around you and extend this feeling further and further to material things around you.

As you breathe in these soft, gentle and heartfelt feelings of gratitude . . . breathing deeply, you relax and feel some tingling chi energy flowing in your spine. Carry on focusing this thanking process by placing your palms as best as you can on any areas of your body which feel panic, fear, pain.

The warmth from your palms seem to penetrate and very soon you start hearing some strange bubbling sounds coming back from that part of your body. Even your head feels lighter and bubbles of gloom and doom may make tiny bursts like soap bubbles popping. (Scientists might prefer to say that the 'synapses are snapping'.)

Follow your breathing. In, pause, out, pause. This time you notice your breath is much deeper. Your breath is much quieter. Your heartbeat has slowed down and feels warmer. You place your hand on your belly and it feels nice, much to your surprise! You feel peaceful. You relax into this deep calm and stillness. You melt into it.

T'ai-Chi – a Rainbow Dance of Nature
You wake up in the morning and you take a walk outside. You see beautiful trees . . . blue sky . . . white fluffy clouds . . . tiny golden flowers on the rich green grass. As you look up from your feet, you see a white dove flying across your path. These visions are in front of you. You are not imagining them.

You can feel the soft breeze . . . the gentle warmth caressing your face . . . as the morning's first rays of sun stream out from behind the clouds bathing your face . . . your whole body is in soft glowing light.

And then, you begin your T'ai-Chi movements. Even if you do not know how to do T'ai-Chi, you feel a stirring of awe and wonder at these majestic visions in front of you. You start to feel that that tree in front of you is you. The branches are your bones, the leaves are your hair, the bark is your skin, the sap is your blood, the roots are your feet. If you had done these movements a thousand times before this moment, they would feel totally different for you right now. You are feeling what the first people who discovered T'ai-Chi felt like 8,000 years ago. Like the tree . . . the wind, the sun's warmth, the birds' songs, your ancient body remembers what that freshness, that aliveness was like. A constant state of release and renewal. Billions of minute muscle cells, blood cells and nerve cells are doing their very best to help you remember this vitality. This message is being circulated throughout your whole body.

Your heart is teaching you how to let go and let it all flow. Each movement is made up of a million or more little movements. A gust of wind passes by and the leaves on the tree wave madly to you. You feel a gush of delight streaming through your body. These tingling sensations are outside as well as inside you. Your face is melting . . . melting into the flowers on that tree . . . melting into the clouds above the tree . . . melting into the green leaves. Your face is a face of faces. These faces of nature are not imagined or painted or designed on paper or canvases. They are constantly changing and cannot be caught by your mind. The faces of Nature belong to Nature. There is absolutely nothing that stands now between your face and the countless myriads of faces of Nature.

Your vulnerability is the vulnerability of Nature. You feel naked inside you. Your mind is aware of unclothing itself from its role plays and responsibilities . . . You feel quiet and silent . . . feeling naked inside. Your heart, body, mind and spirit are open and naked to the whole sky above you.

No drugs, no coffee, no stimulants needed. Just the simplicity of Nature. Every movement in Nature is simultaneously connected to all parts. There is no separation between heart, body, mind and spirit. Any happy or sad experience is felt and accepted. The Heart of the Universe pulsates in the hearts of all. You feel it in the way the sun's rays dance in the rainbow dew-drops on the blades of grass. Happiness is like rays of sunlight bouncing in the eyes of anyone who cares to look. Shimmering golden rainbow lights are everywhere; no matter where you turn, there, the golden colours bounce over to you at the speed of light. You are effortlessly receiving

billions of the most exquisite presents on a day which is not even your birthday.

Today, you can let go of all feelings of inadequacy and worry in the face of this majestic celebration of Nature's colours . . . the breath of innocence in the air. To let yourself go into this lightness and fluidity is so natural because you are naturally a fluid being in your body. A peaceful smile may come up from within you. Let this smile relax your face even more. You can trust the next step . . . the next step . . . Every step feels more and more confident. The smile on your face broadens and broadens and broadens . . . until your smile seem to fill everything. Someone with you may notice your glowing face.

You are the sun's rays from the moment you let go and let the light dance in your whole body. You are the perfume of the flower. You are one with Nature. This is your birthright. This is your priceless gift from Nature in every movement. You are a dancer in the Rainbow T'ai-Chi Dance of Life!

How to appreciate the qualitative beings in yourself and in others
This exercise/principle presents some understanding about how to communicate with nature energy/ light presences. As you move side-ways, going forward and backward, you feel like a carefree child swinging forward and backward in slow motion. In your heart, you

could feel this inner focus of being grateful. Advanced work in this field also uses colours and corresponding qualities to be grateful for. The left side of your body connects to the feminine colours and the right side to the masculine tones.

When you are at the tip-toe part of this exercise, you can connect it to learning to let go, to surrender all those wonderful feelings back to the universal life force. Letting go at the roots of your being.

So, how do we do this? The steps we have taken in other chapters have opened inner doors to a dimension where chi energy is not only experienced but accepted as a fact of Nature. You can experience this especially when you practise T'ai-Chi out of doors, in natural surroundings. Among the natural elements you suddenly feel energizing presences coming through every gesture in your movements, bringing exhilarating sensations throughout your whole being. Gradually, you will get to know them as friends of light and energy presences. You get to communicate with them using a language which they use: colour language.

By visualizing the colours violet, indigo, blue, green, yellow, orange and rose red we are already on the road to meet these presences. There are innumerable hues and shades of all these colours and therefore colour science requires very in-depth, personal study. But the following general ideas can be a starting point for you. They are like learning the ABC of communication with the Nature Light Presences. The best way to understand this is with colour visualization and appreciative sound affirmation, through which you create a balance of Yang and Yin energies. The balance of Yang with Yin attracts the dance of chi energy in you. The dance of Yin and Yang is the dance of Rainbow T'ai-Chi. If you do this consciently, you will experience a oneness with Nature Presences. You will also experience the unconditionally loving and accepting qualities of these colourful and natural presences. Your appreciative affirmations are mirroring back to them what they are. We can discover this only when we follow the advice of a great T'ai-Chi Master: 'Be as humble and as relaxed as a child and you will understand the chi energy.' These Nature Presences exude immense childlike, innocent and pure qualities. There is so much we can learn from them.

Begin by making the following affirmations:

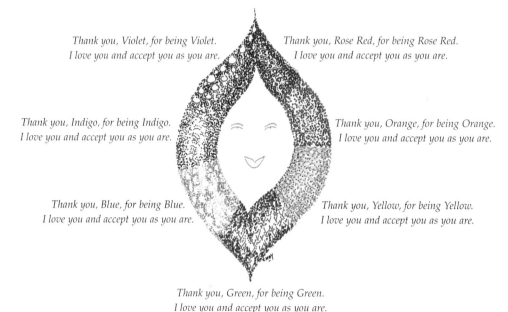

*Thank you, Violet, for being Violet.
I love you and accept you as you are.*

*Thank you, Rose Red, for being Rose Red.
I love you and accept you as you are.*

*Thank you, Indigo, for being Indigo.
I love you and accept you as you are.*

*Thank you, Orange, for being Orange.
I love you and accept you as you are.*

*Thank you, Blue, for being Blue.
I love you and accept you as you are.*

*Thank you, Yellow, for being Yellow.
I love you and accept you as you are.*

*Thank you, Green, for being Green.
I love you and accept you as you are.*

Appreciating the Yin and Yang aspects of colours

After appreciating each colour for its own sake, we go to the next step – appreciating each colour for it Yin/Yang qualities. So now repeat the following affirmations:

*'Thank you, Violet, for being forgiveness and healing light!'
(Visualize healing and forgiving violet light in the hands of healers.)*

*'Thank you, Indigo, for being selfless service and unity in diversity!'
(Visualize an indigo midnight sky like a velvet cloth holding countless unique shiny stars.)*

*'Thank you, Blue, for being peace and clarity!'
(Visualize a clear blue sky with seagulls gliding in the air.)*

*'Thank you, Green, for being harmony and prosperity!'
(Visualize Mother Nature's infinite abundance of greenery in plants, flowers and herbs.)*

'Thank you, Yellow, for being humility, kindness and wisdom!'

(Visualize the golden and radiant faces of the wise men, wise women and wise children.)

*'Thank you, Orange, for being joy and vitality!'
(Visualize the happy smiling faces of children playing in the sun and people drinking revitalizing orange juice on a hot day.)*

*'Thank you, Red, for being love, beauty and courage!'
(Visualize rose red flowers in the hands of someone in love and Red Cross helpers in action.)*

These lists of qualities are based on my research into the many Yin and Yang qualities of colours and applied to every day living. I am sure you will have your own unique experiences and find different meanings for the colours. The list is offered here not as a dogmatic viewpoint but as a starting point for deeper studies into how making friends with colours can improve our lives.

Homework 7

1 Practise the first seven Fundamental T'ai-Chi exercises for 30 minutes every day. Write down any insights.

2 In your own words, what is the Seventh Fundamental Principle/ Dimension?

3 Write down a list of appreciations you can think of about:

a your parents
b yourself in relationship to your job, your appearance, your body, your present situation (whatever this means)
c your partner or close friend(s)

(Note: Initially, this may seem mechanical and unnatural. But with patience and practice, you will start to *feel* it is quite natural rather than having to *think* about it. If you find this difficult, please go back to the first, second and third exercises/ principles .)

4 Do some research into your personal experiences with the world of colours and what they mean for you. Look up different books and research materials on the healing power of colours. Question what you read and put it into practice to see for yourself whether what the experts say is true for you.

To start off, you might want to ask yourself the following questions:

a On occasions when you have a choice, why do you like to wear certain colours? At first the answers may not come. Persevere in your research. Do you see any connection to the colours of Nature and the cycles of the seasons?
b What about the choice of colours of decoration in your home or your own room? How did a certain colour or colour combination affect you or people living with you?
c Flags of nations – can you appreciate how the colours of a flag connect to certain national traits?

Space to record your own insights

_____

_____

_____

_____

_____

☯ *Eighth T'ai-Chi Exercise/Principle*

Dance in your inner fountain of joy!

When to practise
This is a beautiful exercise to do in Nature, facing a tree or at sunrise or sunset.

Best time to practise
In the day time.

Tao of Synthesis
The Real Self blossoms in all its radiance. You are the radiance. You are the centre of that radiance too.

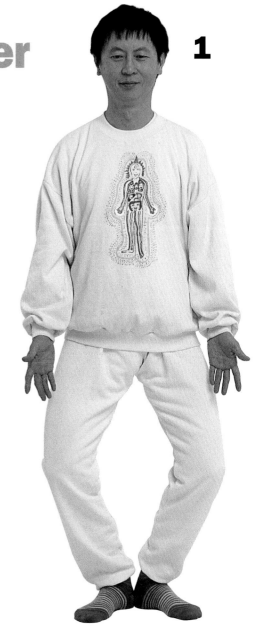

1

1 Stand with your feet in a V-shape, ankle to ankle, at about a 90-degree angle.

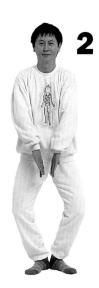

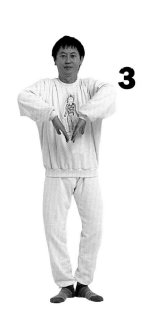

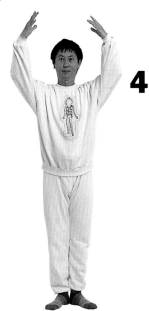

2 Gradually allow your hands to come together between your legs. Your hands touch each other, back to back, with your palms facing outward.

3 Use your elbows to lift your wrists gradually upward. Let your fingers follow your wrists.

4 Your elbows open up to either side of you, like a flower opening her petals. Your fingers follow your elbows by opening upwards, like a fountain of water, as the chi energy shoots gently up from your feet right up to the top of your head.

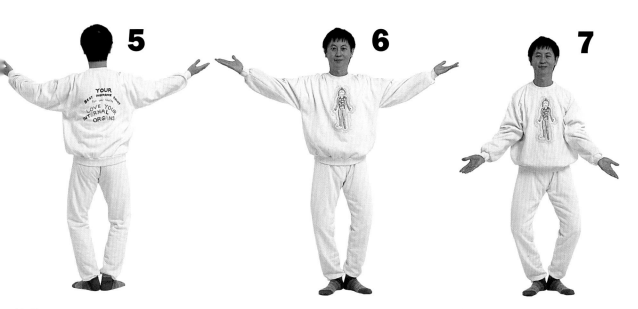

5–7 Your palms open up to face the sky. Now let them fall gently like two leaves descending in slow motion until they drop down to the sides of your body. Gently and gradually move your hands towards the centre in between your legs and begin the whole process again. Do this seven times with all your heart, body, mind and spirit.

'.................... IS ....'

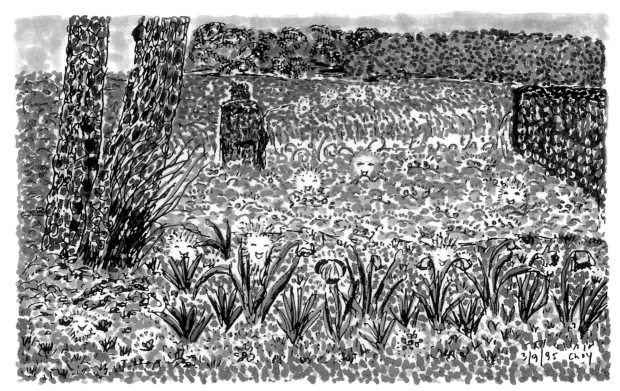

The inner garden of chi
There is, within you, an indescribably beautiful garden and healing waterfall and river of chi energy

This is the eighth dimension, where you discover what your life really is all about. In this dimension you discover that life is because life is. And your whole being is pure energy.

Let us see if we can understand this dimension by looking at the previous steps and then trying to connect to the eighth dimension in the following pages.

The first dimension is about releasing your role plays and responsibilities. Role plays are not bad as long as you can release them. Some people also love certain role plays: but imagine an actor who is playing Macbeth believing he really is Macbeth. When he goes home to his family, he still talks like Macbeth. I recently heard about the father of a T'ai-chi practitioner who is a university lecturer and behaves like a lecturer when he goes home! I know I do it myself – take the job home – and when I realize this, it is time for a good laugh about myself to let go the role play of a T'ai-Chi teacher.

Once you pass through the first dimension, meaning that you are able to release one point of view about yourself or a problem you are facing, you can start to sense the underlying dual nature of the issue in front of you. You see the pros and cons of the issue. And you move into the second dimension. You are able to see two points of view. Your heart feels more balanced and you can accept your own negative and positive reactions towards the situation. The third part of this heart exercise enables you to sow the seed of a third – unknown – possible solution to the problem. And then, as you release it all back to the earth, as the autumn leaves roll back to the earth and are composted into humus, you are willing to trust the earth and beginning to feel that a new spring is coming into your life.

You move on to the next step, into the third dimension. It is a place where you discover that you can see the situation from a non-judgmental point of view, as well as understanding its negative and positive aspects. So, in this sense there are three points of view. In this third dimension, you can love and accept yourself and your situation. You start to realize your underlying search for loving acceptance – your inner child is searching for the love of your inner mother's secure and warm embrace. The embracing of your belly and your chest in this exercise is appropriately designed to remind you that you have the ability to love and accept yourself as you are. You begin to find the beautiful place, where plenitude, peace and love are, as you sink down three times from your knees.

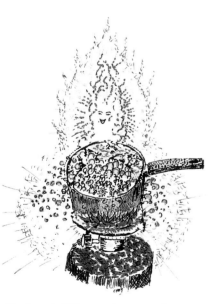

The inner bubbling creative steam of chi energy
Ancient teachers call it kan and li. Let the will of the metal energy create the constructive boundary for the steam of creative pursuits and courageous actions to produce balance – and even a meal or a cup of chi tea!

Many people have heard about 'sinking' in the T'ai-Chi Chuan classics, but they find it difficult to understand what it means in a practical sense. Sinking down into what? Into sorrow? Or into peace, plenitude and loving balance?

As you sink into these beautiful feelings and raise yourself gradually three times from these energies, you begin to sense the fourth dimension coming. The fourth dimension is a place of oneness. A place where there is a natural overflowing. Love smiles in you, bubbling all over you and around you. This loving feeling unifies 'I', 'You' and 'All'. This is the centre of the three steps you have already taken. It can be illustrated as the centre of an equal-sided triangle. The circular nature of the fourth exercise, as your hand moves into a vertical circle, is like a wheel rolling forward and backward. Your inner warmth bubbles up and a boiling point of creativity is reached.

The fifth dimension is inclusive of the four dimensions.

Channel the love from the fourth dimension, not just taking responsibility for our own house, but being aware that whatever each person manifests in his or her life can help to make the planet a better place to live in. It is all ours. Whatever we want is echoed back to us by the universe. A new car, a new house, a loving relationship, etc. The T'ai-Chi boomerang principle. You touch it and let it go. It boomerangs back to you.

Whatever you want will come, at the ripe time. Relax. If you worry about not being able to get what you want

right now, just slide back gracefully into the first, second, third and fourth dimensional steps.

The sixth dimension is about space and lightness.

Emotional space for the best and the worst in you to be accepted exactly as each bit is. Breathing space. Elbow room in your life. Let the lightness come in again with its freshness and spontaneity. Letting go of someone you love very much. Letting go of the pain, too. Releasing and self-acceptance happening together, simultaneously. These qualities of lightness and freedom belong to Beings of Light and Freedom. Inside your body, outside, the whole universe is their playroom.

Enjoy the T'ai-Chi Dance of Space and Light in between your arms, in between your legs, in between your elbows and chest, in between your fingers.

The seventh dimension is about gratitude for the inside and outside. Being grateful for each organ of music in the body, the inner living music that can't be stopped. In the silence of nature, infinite songs of gratitude, suddenly a bird's song may tear into your heart and take you apart into a mad rush of oneness with the universe, appreciating that every moment is beautiful as it is – inside and outside.

And then, a welling up from within, like a fountain of rainbow colours, synthesizing feminine and masculine. You feel all is beautiful. You are happy.

Welcome to the eighth dimension!

The Smiling Chi Fountain Dimension

Imagine a place where your every gesture is a tingling chi movement. It is like being in a sea of energy. The waves of silence are like a billion singing crickets flowing inside you, around you, supporting your hands and feet. Co-ordinated from the centre of your waist, you feel effortless and yet precise. Your whole body glides through the trees, wind, grass, flowers, river, streams, sunlight beams. You feel like a floating bottle of water being uncorked and the inner waters of life join the outer ocean of life. You are one with all life.

Is this all merely imagination?

How do you get to this Smiling Chi Fountain Dimension, bubbling and

The T'ai-Chi Nature Sanctuary
Have you ever sat and sat and sat . . . in front of a growing plant? It can teach you about stillness. You will be able to enter the dimension of smiling chi fountains.

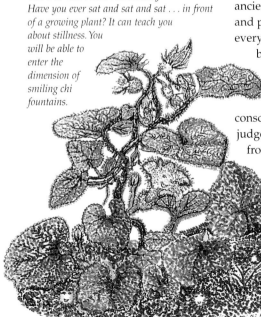

filled with chuckling Light Beings? Where are they? Is it possible to get there?

The answer is, they are inside your body right now. Their messages are in the ancient faces of newborn babies. When you were born, you carried the spirit of the Tao in you. You see in babies that deep, timeless, wise look of a million years. Each baby is unique. When was the last time you saw a tiny baby smile for no particular reason? It is not because you made a funny face. There is an innocent and timeless essence in them radiating a simple message to you. Pure joy is in every creation. The first rays of sunlight falling on a dewdrop. The first songs of the birds to greet the sunlight.

This connection with what the ancient Taoists knew as the pre-birth and post-birth chi is still there inside every nerve cell in your mind and body. This is the inner path in your emotions and mind to the Smiling Chi Fountain Dimension. It is a state of consciousness where there are no judgements; a smile that comes up from your heart where there is a limitless dimension of smiles behind smiles How do you find this dimension? Do you want to go right now? Are you really and sincerely serious about this? If you are truly motivated in your heart, we can do it.

The first step is to slow your mind down and find the path to your heart. Literally. If your mind is not slow enough, you are like an aeroplane soaring through the skies and hoping to smell the fragrance of the flowers on the earth. How do you achieve a quiet mind? First of all, you need to feel that you want to. It may take a number of years. You can study different meditation techniques. Whichever one works for you, practise it. One technique you can practise for about 10-15 minutes a day is to pay attention to the spaces between your thoughts. These inner spaces in your mind allow you to focus on being naturally detached from your thoughts, so that you feel more and more relaxed.

So, let us say you have learned to quieten down your mind. What is the next step?

With a quiet mind, feel yourself gently sinking down into your heart and listening to your heart valves pumping blood around the whole body. Listen to the pulsation of your heart. Feel the pauses in between the heartbeats. You may ask, 'What is the connection between this and the dimension where there are limitless smiles and healing energy?' Well, this exercise of awareness of the heartbeats will open your mind into a spacious dimension. The more you listen to the spaces between your heartbeats, the more receptive you are to these 'limitless spaces'. You are literally touching this limitless space with all your emotion and with all your mind. You feel it and you are being in it now. You are melting into this limitless space. You are this limitless space. Relax into it more and more.

Feeling this limitless, bubbling sense of well-being, naturally you feel grateful to this dimension.

The spaces dance all day and all night. They are bubbling with chi energy right now. Okay, sometimes they play sad music of pain, suffering and abuse. But you realize that you are the new musical director and you can change the tune. You make some wonderful music. You feed your body with new kinds of healthy food for the next seven years. You keep on changing your attitude. You feel lighter, and you feel healthier. Your organs play beautiful songs of inspiration. You may feel inspired to share your energy with others. You feel like painting. You feel like breathing big gulps of happy feelings. You feel on top of your world. You start gardening. You touch everything with tingling chi energy.

What do you want to do? Decorate a room? Decorate it with chi energy. What colours would you like? What colours bring you into a peaceful energy in one room? Visualize that room filled with peaceful energy. Another room brings you into a more loving space. Visualize it filled with loving colours of your choice. Another room you want to make into a place of harmony for meeting friends. And what vibrant colour(s) would you like for your kitchen? Your Smiling Chi Fountain Dimension is a place where chi energy overflows into your living room, your car, your office, your relationship with people, with pets, animals and trees.

When you finish reading or listening to this chapter, take a walk outside and touch everything in your foot-steps with tingling chi energy. In this Smiling Chi Fountain Dimension, you can feel the earth breathe under your feet. Ancient Taoists spoke about the bubbling well under the feet and they meant it literally. You can feel the earth breathe through your feet. You can feel the trees' roots breathing through your feet. You will naturally feel a sense of rootedness and limitless peace in your daily movements. In fact, they feel more and more like your T'ai-Chi movements. When you feel nervous in your stomach, you will turn to the inner sanctuary in your tan-tien centre for confidence and you will learn to trust your chi energy reservoir to supply your nervous self with confident feelings of nourishment. When you feel worry in your spleen – or if you just feel worried and you are not even sure which part of you feels anxious – turn within this gentle space and feel chi energy calming you and allowing you to realize chi is there with whoever you are worried about.

In this quiet space, smiles of all kinds bubble up. There are peaceful smiles, loving smiles, joyous, laughing smiles, healing smiles, smiling harmony and beautiful smiling feelings. Breathe. Take a pause. Take another pause . . . Breathe. Feel this inner space stretch in your consciousness beyond your physical body. Expand your awareness to the horizons. Let your awareness go beyond the chair or bed or whatever physical thing is supporting you right now. Let your awareness go beyond the roof tops, the sky, the earth . . . right now. Your smiles expand and expand and expand. The lighter you are, the more you are open to chi energy. Chi can only flow, flower and bubble up in you when you are vibrating with a finer and purer and purer vibration. So, how do you get into this purer and purer vibration?

The ancient Taoists say, 'Smile gently to every cell in your whole body.'

Every cell in your body is a smiling cell. The lightness in you frees every cell in your body, especially those parts that feel heavy, tired or in pain. Feel the light pulsating, spreading and filling every cell with lightness right now. Discomfort is the body's way of telling you it is in need of limitless rejuvenating and healing chi. Where do you get this chi? From limitless chi in this limitless space. Feel every cell opening to receive limitless rejuvenating and healing chi. Feel all your organs returning to healthy function.

Limitless chi is vibrating in every cell right now. Limitless chi is here right now . . . Breathe it. Can you feel it? Breathe in . . . pause . . . breathe out. Feel limitless space in your breath. Feel your breath melting into limitless space. Breathe in . . . breathe out. Breathe in . . . breathe out.

Relax, deeper and deeper into this tingling energy.

Feel all your organs feeling this chi energy right now. Tingling warm chi vibrating. All organs returning to normal healthy function. Your organs are organs of symphony. They play the most exquisite music of harmony within you when you are well. Visualize your organs vibrant with chi. They are well and healthy right now. They sing. They play.

Chi energy, light and warmth
What is the relationship between chi energy and the essence of water, light and warmth? As water quenches our thirst, so do the combined sparkling essences of chi-filled water, light and warmth quicken this rejuvenation process for your whole being. Then you start seeing psychic lights, colours and spiritual presences.

During these moments you may feel you are being swept off your feet. You need to keep doing your T'ai-Chi and Chi Kung exercises in order to remain grounded. You may also start to familiarize yourself with the energy as coming from a specific source, and then you start to recognize it (from past associations) as coming from a set of symbols, formulas and person(s). And when you learn to set aside your past associations of chi energy, you cognize (that is, you know directly without preconceived ideas) it. Chi can express itself through limitless forms and does not need our past experiences to give it reality.

The best place to continue this practice of cognizing chi is within you right now. There is light, warmth and fluidity within your body. Without the inner light of consciousness you could not see in your dreams or even think of the

At the end of your Rainbow T'ai-Chi practice, golden radiant energies of abundant health are awaiting you.

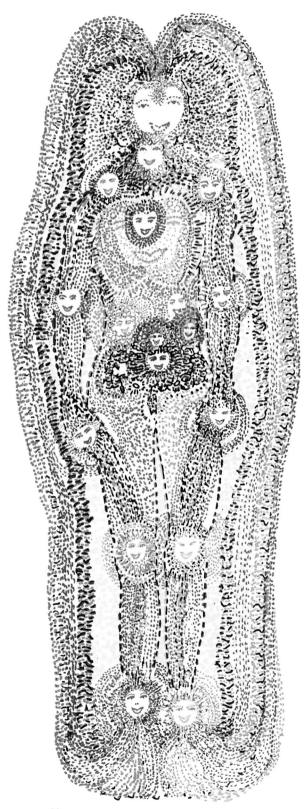

question, 'Where is the loo?' The body's natural warmth and fluidity is the best place for you to test how chi relates to the essence of water, light and warmth. Feel it energize your internal organs, starting from your heart. There is this pulsating warmth not just inside your heart but also on your chest. At first it is just a gentle stirring of warmth, like a little budding flower opening her petals. As you watch it with gentle respect and gratitude, it grows and glows into a flower of shining warmth and light. Let its radiance extend beyond the horizons of your body, of the room. Go beyond the house, the planet . . . the sky.

In this Smiling Chi Fountain Dimension, you can feel chi energy enlivening every creative project in your life right now. Whatever you have set your heart on achieving, chi will help you achieve it. This is not simply a strong desire – literally your heart is there with you every step along the way. Taoists believe that the heart is the governor of the internal organ systems. Silently affirm this within you right now, with real loving tenderness, as your heart is doing her very best to carry life-supporting energy and nutrients to every cell in your whole being.

Feel your gratitude flowing through your blood vessels. Feel your immune system strengthening with every passing second. Feel your nervous system empathizing with your endeavour right now. You are endeavouring to send a message of limitless support to your muscular system, so that it goes one hundred per cent to do whatever needs to be done to achieve your projected creative goals in your life right now.

Right now there are marvellous little paths of light and energy all over you – inside and outside. They have been there always. The ancient sages gave them names as acupuncture meridians and channels. At the ripe time, through more years of advanced practice, you will discover how the Yin and Yang meridians of energies flow together in the fifteen ways to find an even happier you.

As these healing energies increase in intensity, you will naturally connect with the five elements of Nature – water, air, wood, metal and earth. This interconnectedness has always been there.

Chi energy and water
How do you relate to water in your everyday life when you are filled with chi awareness? In the dimension of chi, the ancients thought of water as having an essence of its own. As you melt further and further into it, it could be translated into a water-like state of being. As you make friends with this 'spirit of water', it shares secrets of rejuvenation and youth with you. The water you drink, the water you bathe in, the water you cook and wash with, the rivers and swimming pools you swim in are charged with chi energy.

Chi energy and air
As you keep feeling this radiant chi pulsating from your heart and around you . . . breathe in the chi, feel it energizing even more the physical cells in your body. As you breathe out, feel it pulsating in your blood, flowing through your lungs. The air you breathe in and out is charged with chi. Breathe in . . .feel the chi . . . breathe out . . . pause . . .

feel the chi . . . breathe in. Feel millions of sparkling streams of chi flowing through your blood vessels, throughout your whole body. Every cell is a cell of energy. And it is there ever ready for you. (You have a limitless supply of energized Eveready batteries within you!)

Chi energy and tan-tien
In your belly centre, chi gathers into a large pool. That is how the name 'tan-tien' came about. It literally translates as 'sea of chi energy.' Like a molten sun-like essence, your tan-tien shines and radiates health.

Chi energy, wood and metal
Every item you eat contains elements of plants and metals. Chi energizes all these elements when your body transforms them into useful nutrients that can be easily assimilated for use or for storage in your organs. All your organs are shining with immense delight and chi. Not only are they your amazing, miraculous workers of transformation and tireless servers, but they too can receive limitless gratitude from you right now. And they shine back to you with gratitude. Billions of 'thank you' messages carried by billions of nerve cells are bouncing to and fro between every organ in your body.

Chi and the earth
As you collect more chi energy in your tan-tien, it naturally overflows and energizes your internal organs even more. Chi also flows down your legs and connects to the earth, like the roots of a tree spreading deep down to the centre of the earth. Feel chi radiantly touching the essence of the earth too. Just as you may sense colourful beings when your chi touches the elements of

light, warmth, water and air, you may see visions of colourful beings in the earth, too. Wherever you walk, you can feel chi and gratitude pulsating through your feet. You can exchange beneficial and healthy radiant energy with the earth.

With our head in the sky and our feet rooted to the earth, we can make the earth a sanctuary, a place filled with chi energy, a place for healing and rejuvenation. You may think that this sounds like an impossible task. On the other hand you never know – one day, this wish might come true. Every journey begins with one step. And that step can be taken from your own doorstep. You make this step into yourself. The best place to begin is inside you. Wherever you go, you take you with you. You are this T'ai-Chi Natural Sanctuary. Fill you with chi. The elements of Nature are in you. And generations after you will follow you. In their own unique ways, they will generate chi and allow chi to express itself through limitless ways. And one day, the earth will be populated with chi-energized and chi-conscious people. There are already more than 10 million people – yes, right this moment, even as you are reading or listening to this book – working silently to bring chi into their bodies and allow chi to feel at home. Your organs can truly be a home for chi. We have returned home to chi. Chi is our basic nature.

Homework 8

1 Do the eight Fundamental T'ai-Chi exercises and explain in your own words what the eight Fundamental T'ai-Chi principles are.

2 Jot down any inspiring encounters you have with Light Beings. Do not worship or denounce these experiences. One day they may make some sense to you.

3 Draw parts of your body that you have difficulty loving and in your drawing surround them with loving light. See your whole body – every organ, tendon, muscle and cell – as being radiant with light. Realize every day that prosperity and health are synonymous.

4 Visualize every single thing you see in front of you – furniture, pencil, typewriter, vacuum cleaner, etc. – as being filled with minute as well as immense energizing light beings.

5 Connect the 'I am love, you are love, all is love' chant to touch every single thing you can think of and every feeling you can feel inside and outside you. (Do this chanting inwardly if you do not want to disturb people around you.) Let everything be touched by the sound of the light and love within you.

6 Record any insights from these chanting and light visualization exercises.

Space to record your own insights

_____

_____

_____

_____

_____

_____

_____

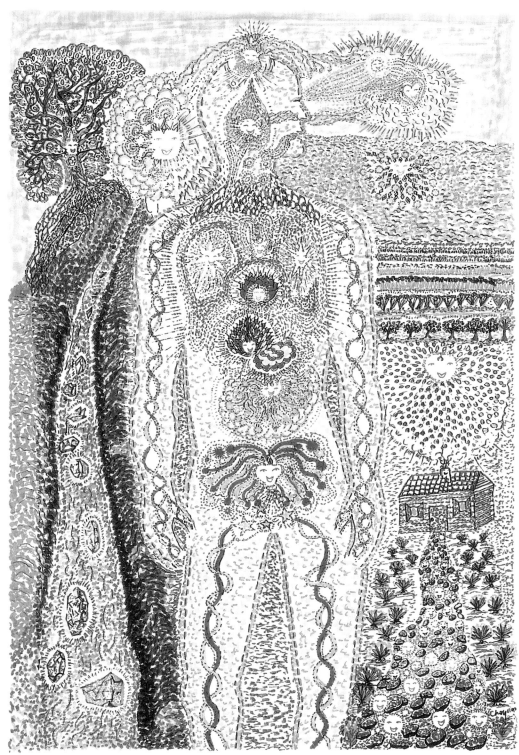

*Rainbow T'ai-Chi
Man*
*Rainbow T'ai-Chi is
the discovery of the
Rainbow River of
Qualities which flow
within our bodies and
in our daily life.*

☯ First Chi Kung Exercise/Principle
Harmonize your inner feminine/ masculine/creative aspects

When to practise
Practise this exercise/principle when you feel afraid, insecure or lonely, and when you feel in need of extra chi energy.

Best time to practise
Pick a quiet time in the night when the neighbours and everyone in your house are asleep, or close yourself in a room away from other people.

Tao of Green Lessons
Learn to grow like the roots of a tree. With infinite patience, hope and trust in nourishing chi, the true purpose of your life unfolds step by step before your very eyes. Learn to look for the steps of progress you are making now if you want to find out what is in store for you in the future.

This Chi Kung exercise connects with the Yin, Yang and Tao, which correspond to the inner feminine/motherlike, the inner masculine/fatherlike and creative/childlike aspects of ourselves.

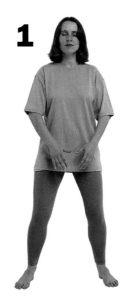

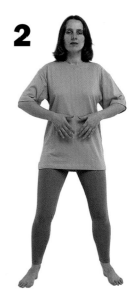

1–2 With palms open, feel and visualize an inner child in your belly centre, embraced in warmth and gentle nourishment. Slowly bring your hands from below, feeling the earth's forces going up into your belly. As the earth nourishes you with all her wealth of food, water and materials to keep you sheltered and cared for, you can touch your inner child with this powerful feeling from the earth. Allow

the warmth from your palm to embrace your inner child and let your palms stay on your belly area for a few seconds. (When you feel nervous, afraid or anxious, your belly feels as if butterflies were flapping away inside it, because of your lack of self-confidence, your feeling of not being good enough. Stay in this centre and be with this frightened and insecure inner child until he or she is calm.)

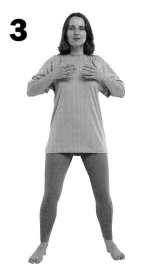

3

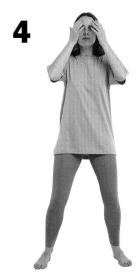

4

3 After about 1–3 minutes of connecting with your inner child in your belly, gently move your hands up, passing your diaphragm and moving slowly towards your heart region. Place both palms on your chest. This Chi Kung position of crossed hands on your chest connects to your feminine aspect, the picture of your inner mother/woman, the part of you which sometimes feels trapped in different roles and responsibilities (as a house-wife, mother, lover, etc.). For a man, it could also connect to your inability to express feelings of hurt by crying. If you feel this inability now, touch your chest, your heart, your life with a new feeling of tenderness, a new feeling of inner embrace. Instead of depending on the outside for approval and the warmth, you can turn inward and share this inner warmth with yourself and your loved ones. From the chi energy level, your embrace is timeless.

4 Now, from your heart area, let your palms move up, passing your throat to face your eyes. Keep your palms still in front of your eyes for a minute. Allow their warmth to relax your eye muscles and facial muscles. Visualize a masculine image of yourself – independent, bright and courageous.

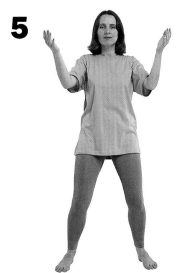

5

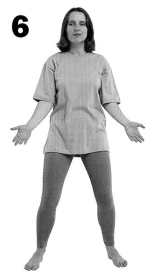

6

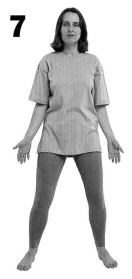

7

5 Open your palms and feel your mind open and free.

6–7 Allow your arms and palms to fall gently to your sides. Open your palms and allow them to float down in slow motion, like leaves from a tree. Feel your palms falling in a zig-zag motion as the air seems thicker and thicker, supporting the fall of your hands. You can feel that your hands are supported and cushioned by the air underneath. Let your feet sink and root into the earth. Return to the original position and start all over again.

Taking heartfelt steps in your life

Homework 9

Imagine a day when whatever you do, you do it from an inner sense of harmony and peace. You have made the decision to feel caring and with your whole being you have decided to look for the best, and to appreciate what you find.

Each passing second, 2 million new mature red blood cells enter your circulation to maintain normal blood supply in your whole body. Isn't that an amazing thing, and something to give thanks for?

When you step on the pavement ready to go to work, every cubic millimetre of your footstep has more than 5 million red blood cells, totally supporting you.

Even though you may not be aware of it, your heart is pumping blood at 75 beats per minute, carrying precious nourishment to your whole body and helping to get rid of wastes. What an incredible

miracle the heart organ is, isn't it? From your heart, feel your chi energy flow within your blood, carrying billions of messages of appreciation to every cell.

Feel this in your arms, your hands, your neck, your legs.

Feel harmony in the way your feet are moving.

Feel peace in the way your heart pulsates.

Feel chi energy through your whole body.

Throughout your life and your parents' lives, you as a child and parent will always receive an abundance of harmony and peace in your body. Even when you are unwell, your body does its very best to keep on caring.

In your heart, you know this to be true.

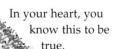

The Light Being in your heart

1 Practise this exercise for about 15 minutes a day. Record any insights.

2 In your own words, what is the purpose of the First Chi Kung Exercise/Principle?

3 How do you understand the Yin/feminine, Yang/masculine and Tao/creative principles as they relate to Nature's elements?

4 How is this connected to a having a greater awareness of your own inner child, mother and father aspects?

5 Describe your past childhood, teenage and adult development in terms of your challenge to find a more balanced Yin/feminine/loving, Yang/masculine/clarifying and Tao/creative/playful lifestyle. Give examples of some of these challenges.

6 Describe as best as you can your parents' situation in terms of their balance or imbalance of Yin/ feminine/loving, Yang/masculine/ clarifying and Tao/creative/playful attitudes and activities.

7 List the qualities of the inner mother, inner father and inner child you would like to have in yourself. Reflect on what kind of activities/ courses/projects would be useful to help remind you of these inherent natural qualities.

How the Inner Family Chi Kung exercise worked miracles for Paul's health and business challenges

It was Paul's second session. He had been practising the Chi Kung exercise to connect his inner child, mother and father.

When he came for his first two-hour session a week ago, he had complained of tiredness and difficulty in breathing. He said he felt emotionally unstable and easily got impatient, intolerant and angry with his co-workers and his family. Today, when he touched his belly, he connected to his inner child and felt some pain.

Paul shared, 'When I was a little boy, I was punished a lot for misbehaving. I felt fearful about going home. When I dirtied my school uniform, even though it was only a raincoat, I tried to throw it away, but my parents found out where I hid it and I got a "hiding". I was not supposed to cry when I got the beatings. I was convinced that I deserved it. I held back my tears. I learned to control my feelings and suppress all my emotions inside me. Whenever I went home I felt inadequate, not good enough.'

The First Chi Kung Exercise enabled Paul to get in touch with this past aspect of himself, an aspect which was still very much in him. He saw how his attitude to parental authority still lived in him psychologically in his role as a boss; the way he treated people around him was like the way his parents treated him. Gradually he started letting go and the tears flowed.

Paul gave all his attention in this exercise to his inner child, placing his palms on his belly and learning how simply to be there with his inner child's pain. 'I was naughty in order to get some attention,' he said, on behalf of his inner child. His palm felt warm on his belly. He had always enjoyed being around people and as a child he liked to play games This aspect had stayed in him and could be seen even in his present job. For the past ten years he had been running a leisure centre, but for the past six years he had worked from early morning till eleven o'clock at night and had not taken even a day off with his family. His wife also worked long hours, like him.

After a week of practising the Chi Kung exercise at least twice a day, every day, Paul came to see me and shared that he felt much more relaxed and that his breathing had improved tremendously.

He also shared that on the way to see me, he had had an inspiration. For him, it was like a miracle. Not only had he slowed down his mind and feelings, he had come up with a real solution to his problem. Instead of working such long hours, he was going to work harder for fewer hours and earn more. His sense of economizing effort was apparent in the relaxed way he moved his arms and body. There was a much more concentrated awareness in the way he moved. And this economical, concentrated awareness gave him a similar awareness of how to reorganize his own business. He told me he would also have more time in the evenings to relax.

I asked him, 'How does your inner child feel about this idea?' He placed his palms on his belly and silently attuned within for a couple of minutes. Then he beamed, 'He is jumping about and feeling happy!' What about his inner mother? Again, a short pause as he closed his eyes to look inside and ask her. 'She says she will have more time to spend with me. My inner father said that he liked the idea because he will have more time to be interested in me.' Paul then shared how his physical family would also be pleased with this news. He used the Chi Kung exercise to open up not only his negative feelings of repressed anger, but also some joyful moments from his childhood. He connected to how his inner child's happy and 'full of stamina' days – playing football, for example – contained the same feelings as his parents experienced in their own ways.

There is a Paul inside all of us, waiting to be discovered. We have hidden treasures, and no amount of 'hiding' can take those miraculous inner treasures from us. It is our inherited treasury of peace, joy, timeless patience and love. We have only to slow down, touch those deep aspects of our being and truly feel at home with ourselves. This is the real miracle that happened for Paul.

☯ Second Chi Kung Exercise/Principle
For uplifting your spirit

When to practise
When you feel depressed, unappreciated and uninspired in your relationship or job. Practise it also when you want to experience more prosperity and health in your life.

Best time to practise
Out of doors with your head looking at an open blue sky and your feet firmly on the ground.

Tao of Blue lessons
Learn to reach for the highest within you. You are like a unique star shining your blue light of deep calmness and clarity on to troubled areas in your life.

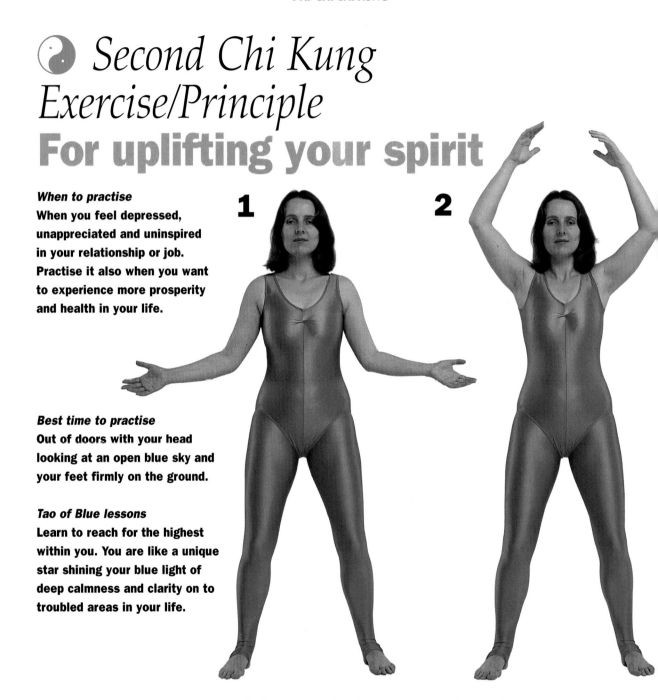

1–2 Start in a relaxed posture with your knees bent and your feet about shoulder-width apart. Allow your hands to lift up from your sides, gradually and slowly, with your palms facing upwards.

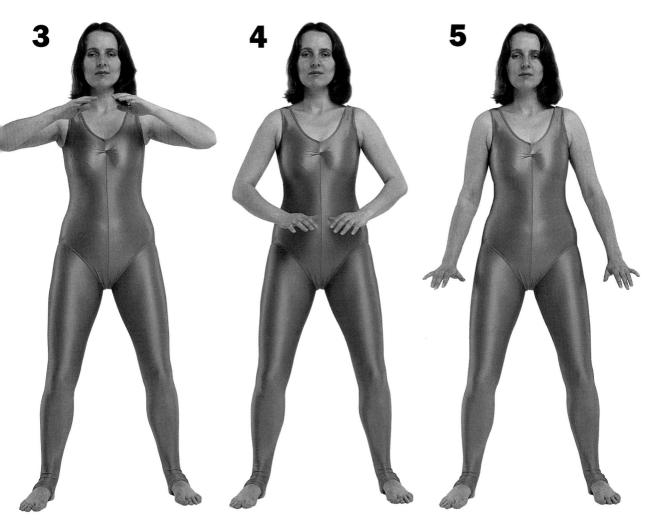

3 Lift your arms up above your head until the palms are facing each other. As your arms rise, think of an uplifting and inspiring experience.

4 As you allow your arms to sink slowly down towards the earth, with your fingertips together and palms down, think of activities (such as gardening, walking, etc.) which help you feel grounded.

5 Let your hands drop towards your belly centre. Feel yourself rooting into the earth like a tree.

Your happiness does not need to depend on the external

Homework 10

Feel uplifted as your arms rise up. Breathe in at the same time. You have the power to inspire yourself. Let smiles of gratitude bubble up from within you.

When you look at a baby smiling, can you feel how effortless it is? This baby smile could be for a complete stranger, passing by on a bus or outside a shop. It is like a ray of sunshine that breaks through the hectic speed and sometimes hard and bitter aspects of the adult world we live in. For a few moments, we are uplifted. But how did that smile do that? Did that baby know you from some past life? You are not sure. Does it really matter? The fact is you feel uplifted. The smile is not there because you have done some good deed. It is not there because it is your birthday or because you have gained some special promotion in your job. The smile is simply there. And if you let it in, it transforms you. It makes you feel glad and grateful for babies. This effortless smile is still inside you.

So why do you not feel it if it is inside you? You can only rediscover this smile when you return to that non-judgmental smiling state (see page 80). And it is there. It is pure and cannot be polluted by the fears and pain created by the adult mind. It is not created by the adult mind. This eternal reminder is in every cell of your body. As every cell is effortlessly and non-judgmentally released and new radiant cells are being born in your bone marrow, the body naturally radiates a smile of health. It is already within you, within your body.

Read the following and then, if you would like to, close your eyes. Look inside you, into your tan-tien centre. Relax into the stillness. When you meditate and melt into this stillness, you will naturally feel a peaceful smile coming up. Feel uplifted by this smile. Feel it flower in your whole being. Feel it bubble up like an ever-expanding smile. Feel it filling your whole consciousness. Let yourself melt into it and become 'unconscious'. Then, without your even being aware of it consciously, someone may remark that you look beautiful and that you have a face like a lovely baby!

And so, when you do this Chi Kung movement, your face will naturally feel different. As your arms rise up, let your inner radiant smile shine bright and strong, like waves of the sun's rays bouncing from the earth back to the heavens. As your arms sink back towards the earth through the middle section of your body, let the chi energy from the heavens pour right through you. Spirals of energy flowing through your movement: 'May the Heavens smile upon you.'

1 Practise this exercise for about 15 minutes a day. Write down your insights.

2 In your own words, what is the purpose of this Second Chi Kung Exercise/Principle?

3 Describe what you think or feel chi energy is. What happens to a part of your body when it is energized with chi? (Note: If there is any physical injury to any part of your body, in addition to any other forms of treatment you may be using, place your palm above the affected part and allow chi to help accelerate the body healing process. Record your daily observations of how chi helps the body to heal at a natural pace.)

4 Think of some activities/interests that were meaningful for you when you were a child. What did you like to do or play with?

5 Think of ten activities/interests in your present life which uplift you.

6 Think of ten activities/interests which help you feel grounded.

Space to record your own insights

☯ *Third Chi Kung Exercise/Principle*
Purify and recycle your energy through your kidneys
Part One

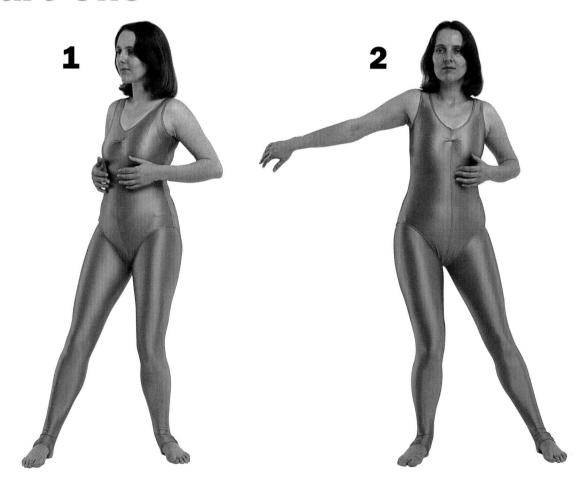

1–3 With your feet parallel and about shoulder-width apart, place your palms on either side of your abdomen. Be still for a minute. In the stillness, visualize your palms gently holding

your kidneys. Feel the tingling warm chi nurturing your kidneys. Feel tingling warmth from your palms relaxing your kidneys.

Shift your weight on to your left leg and turn your waist and right arm to your right. Slowly and gently throw your arm back, then bring it to the front again (as in the Second

When to practise
When you feel lacking in vitality and off-centred, you need the help of your kidneys and heart to find vitality and balance again.

Best time to practise
At night or whenever you have some quiet time so you can really tune in to your organs. When you go on holiday by the sea, do it in front of the waves – a truly amazing experience!

Tao of Blue lessons
Flow with life and life flows with you. Become a swimmer in chi energy. The world is your swimming pool.

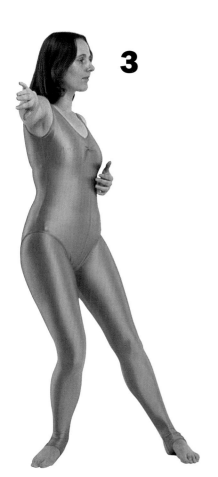

3

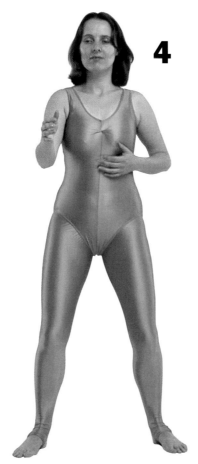

4

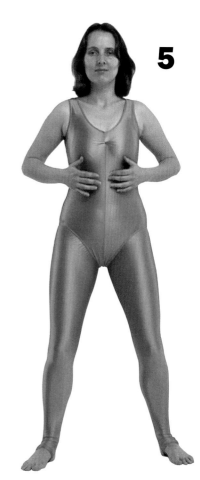

5

Fundamental Tai-Chi Exercise, page 30) and turn your waist so that you are facing to the left with your arm stretched out in front of you.

4 Gradually twist your wrist and let your palm float down slowly and gently as you turn your waist to face forwards again. Twist and sink your elbow gently down towards your right kidney area.

5 Now, bring your palm towards the front, back to the starting position. Repeat the exercise on the other side in exactly the same way.

Part Two

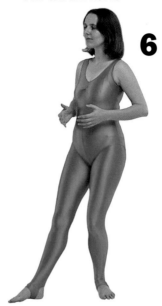

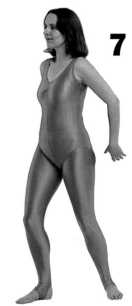

6 Start by placing both palms on your kidneys and shift all your weight to your left foot. Take a slow and deliberate step forward with your right foot so that it is at an angle of about 45 degrees to the left foot.

7 Move your arms gently to your sides and extend both your lower arms behind you like a swimmer about to dive into a pool. Gradually shift your weight forward as you move your arms in front of you.

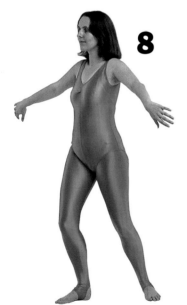

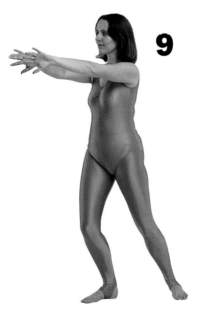

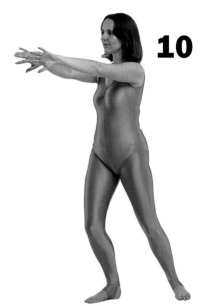

8–9 Allow your little fingers to point upwards as you gently raise your arms

so that your hands come together, back to back.

10 Now, turn your elbows and sink them down towards the ground.

Part Three

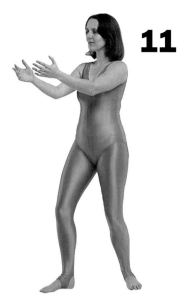

11

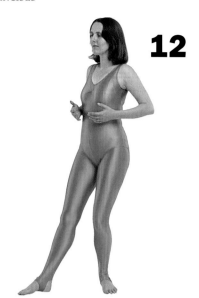

12

11 Gradually draw your palms towards your kidneys. As you do this, shift your weight back on to your left leg. Your palms should now be close to your kidneys.

12–13 Sink your palms down below your waist in front of your lower abdomen. It is as if your palms were tracing the urinary tubes (ureters) to the region in front of your bladder. With your palms moving parallel to each other, shift your weight forward again on to your

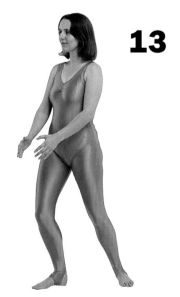

13

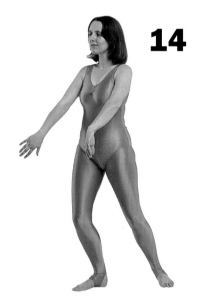

14

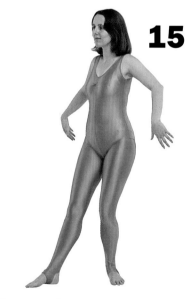

15

right foot. Make sure your elbows stay close to your diaphragm and are not overstretched. An ideal angle between lower and upper arm is about 100 degrees.

14–15 Open your palms to the sides and turn them around behind you in a circular way. Bring your palms back in front of your kidneys again.

Now repeat Steps 6–15.
Then do the whole exercise on the other side, with the left foot out.

You can learn from your kidneys to filter and clean up your past and release the old, recycling the best

Your kidneys are located just inside your lower ribs, at the back of your body. When you touch the front of your body opposite that point, you will be able to feel your kidneys. Imagine your palms are inside your body, touching your kidneys with the utmost care and gentleness. For many people, feeling the kidneys is a soft, warm, spongy sensation. You feel more balanced, with a sense of fullness and energy. Your whole body is glowing, and this shows on your face, too.

Gently place your palms on your kidneys for a minute and then lift them a few inches away from your body. Feel the space under your palms warm and tingling. Patiently be with this warmth for about 5 minutes. Let your palms touch and then let go again. Touch and then let go again. Imagine that you can go in and touch your kidneys, feel them, feel the soft and spongy feeling there. How would you hold your only pair of kidneys, if you were able to? Feel your caring and gently rhythmic palms moving in small circles, massaging your kidneys with chi energy and warmth. Appreciate them for all the years of selfless service they have given you. Your kidneys help you to clean and purify your blood.

A lot of memories of hurt, pain and pleasure are not properly digested and assimilated. Please look up other exercises, particularly the Second T'ai-Chi Exercise and Principle (page 30) for more details about how to digest and assimilate your past. In this Kidney Chi Kung Exercise, you can also be aware that you are taking in your whole past, accepting responsibility for the purification of those hard-won experiences and sifting them to find the golden, loving feelings behind them.

When you feel intensely afraid, you may feel it affect even your kidneys. It is like a child being afraid to ask the teacher for permission to go to the toilet – he or she just sits there, holding it all in. Whenever I do workshop sessions on the subject of fear, I notice that people suddenly get up to visit the toilet more than usual! But behind the fearful memories there exists the side of you that desires security, comfort and love. This side comes out more strongly when fear is around; fear acts as a catalyst to attract qualities of courage, balance, gentleness and kindness. You can feel this awareness of courage, balance, gentleness and kindness when you do this exercise of moving out. This clarification process is sensing, 'Every negative brings us to a greater positive and creative balance!' You may find it useful to repeat this affirmation when you feel acute fears coming on. Do the Kidney Chi Kung Exercise in your imagination, if you cannot find the space to do it physically.

When your palms go forward (the 'diving palms' part), you can feel yourself releasing the old experiences, just as your kidneys release the waste urea through your

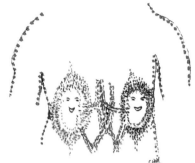

Visualization for the Kidney Chi Kung Exercise
Being kind to the internal organs is a very important part of 'Chi Kung for health' practice

ureter tubes to your bladder. You could enjoy this release or think of it as a waste of time. Next time you urinate, ask yourself if you are present for this part of your daily life, or if are you wishing it all to be over quickly (and sometimes painfully if you have kidney trouble such as kidney stones). Is your consciousness present for this amazing skill that life has taught you? You can feel grateful and appreciate the marvellous sensation of release fully.

Many people call this movement a 'swimming in the air' sensation, as you join the 'diving palms' experience with the 'diving arms' exercise. The more you do this exercise, the thicker and heavier the air feels. You will feel more relaxed and peaceful and some people even sweat, although they have not done any hard physical exercise. The sweat glands are connected to the urinary system. As your chi circulation improves in your kidneys, the same 'clearing out' signals will spread throughout your body.

Homework 11

1 Practise both the single- and the double-handed movements of this exercise with the First and Second Chi Kung Exercises, for about 30 minutes a day. Record any insights.

2 In your own words, explain the purpose of the Third Chi Kung Exercise/Principle.

3 The filtering/cleansing principle of this exercise is connected to your daily life. How are the Yin/Yang and Tao principles reflected in the functions of the vacuum cleaner, the washing machine and the dishwasher (if you have them)?

4 The balancing principle of the exercise also connects to balance in your diet. You might be interested to do some research into balancing your diet and finding out which types of foods correspond to the five elements (see page 83) and the five tastes of Chinese tradition. Here is a starting point of enquiry:

Five elements diet
Wood – sour taste affecting the liver/gall bladder;
Fire – bitter taste affecting the heart/small intestine;
Earth – sweet taste affecting the spleen/stomach;
Metal – spicy/pungent taste affecting the lungs/large intestine;
Water – salty taste affecting the kidneys and bladder.

5 There is also a need to balance the energy-reducing foods, which are Yin/cool/cold, with energy-producing foods which are Yang/warm/hot. Can you name some foods which fit into these categories?

6 Which acidic foods (some examples are alcohol, bread, cheese, coffee, fruit juices, meat, salad dressings, tea) and which alkaline foods (baked potatoes, green vegetables and grains) do you like?

Space to record your own insights

☯ *Fourth Chi Kung Exercise/Principle* **Spring**

1

2

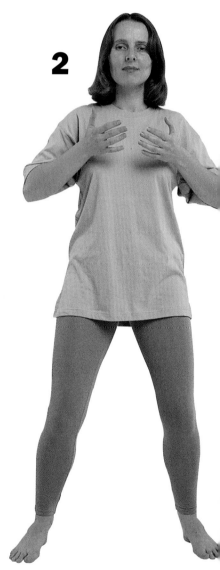

When to practise
When you are starting on new projects, ideas and inspirations. When you wake up in the morning or when you have been sitting at your desk too long with your shoulders drooping – you can open up your chest and breathe.

Best time to practise
Any time during the day. Make sure you have space to either side of you so that you can stretch.

Tao of Green lessons
When it is the ripe time to let your ideas sprout, be tender, as a mother naturally is with her newborn babe.

1 With feet parallel and about shoulder-width apart and knees bent, gradually move your hands to the sides of your thighs. Bring your palms up gently, feeling the chi energy moving up your legs towards your tan-tien centre. Then, feel as if you were lifting something up.

2 Bring your palms up to the area in front of your chest.

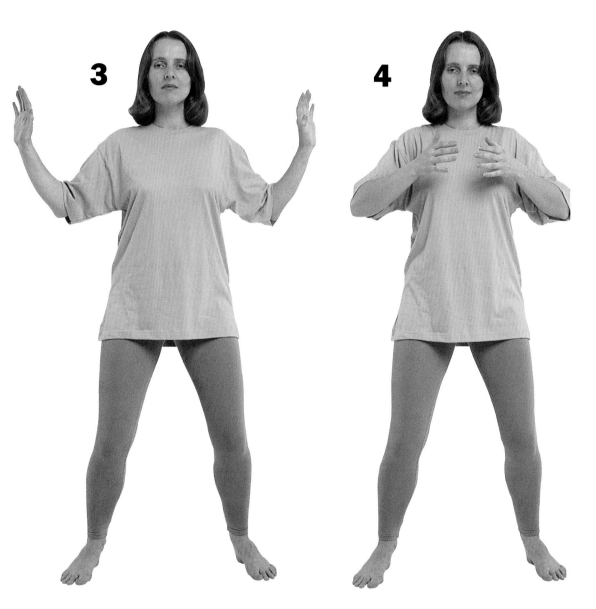

3 Turn your wrists from your elbows towards your chest and push out gently to the sides. Bend your elbows and keep them sunk as you push your palms out. Let your hands come up as if you are pushing against a wall on either side of you.

4 Gradually bring your hands back to your chest area.

Fifth Chi Kung Exercise/Principle Summer

When to practise
Whenever you feel unsure and too serious about your life.

Best time to practise
Out of doors on a bright sunny day.

Tao of Yellow lessons
Be as the Laughing Buddha, holding up the bright sunny sky above his head. Wisdom is based on the balance between intuitive action, the ability truly to hear others and the ability to remain grounded in common sense.

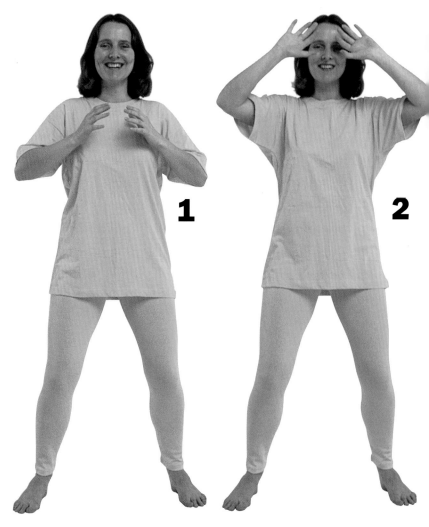

1 Starting from the point in the Spring exercise (page 100–101) where your palms are pushed out, gradually bring your palms back to the chest area.

2 Turn your palms upwards and outwards, lifting your head slightly to look up.

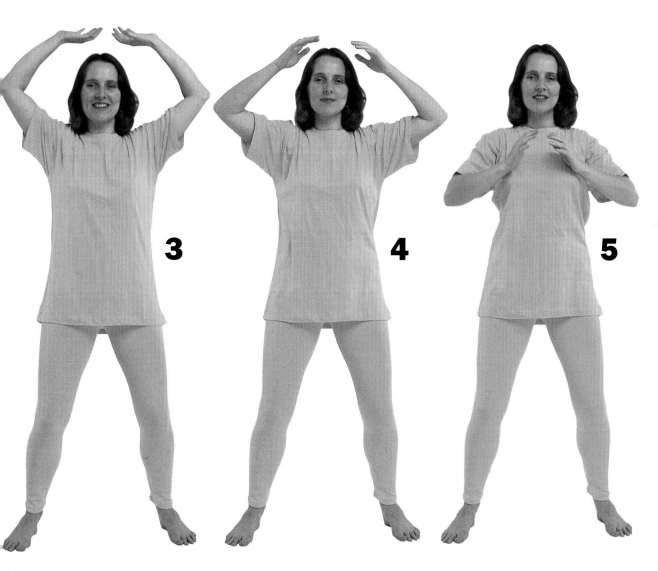

3 Push your arms up so that they form an arch. Feel your palms holding something up there. Some Chi Kung Masters call this the 'holding of the heavens' posture.

4–5 Gradually bring your hands back to the chest area.

Giving birth to the new in your life

When you first do the Spring Chi Kung Exercise, you may feel a little unsure and perhaps even judgmental of yourself. When you learn to let go of the judging aspect of the Yang self in you and flow more easily with the movements, you begin to feel the lighter aspect of the Yang self. You feel calmer and more confident.

This calmness and confidence can gradually grow into a seed of purity and innocence in you. Seed projects in your daily life flourish from your calmness and confidence. It may take some slow, gentle and intense focus, feeling the space between your palms and the physical space, but you will get there.

This new, confident part of yourself is like a new spring, a new river springing up from the ground. An inner smile bubbles up innocently like the smile of a baby, from your tan-tien centre, moving towards your heart, a feeling of release, opening you up. You are like a little seedling plant opening its first new leaves, thrusting out of the fertile soil of your imagination to greet the sunny blue sky of opportunity.

Free, free at last! Your time to live, to go all out to achieve what you want from your life is here now!

Relationship and business challenges become creative opportunities to grow and to understand yourself better. Your mistakes are no longer regarded as 'bad', merely as steps to enable you to grow. Your self-awareness exercises become effective, practical ways of improving your daily achievements. New angles of looking at old problems appear to you. You are opening yourself up to new enthusiasms, new inspirations, new ideas and new vitality all the time.

Growing and celebrating the best in you

In this Summer Chi Kung movement (pages 102–103), you melt into a heightened sense of creativity – joy in action! Just as Nature flowers and bears fruits, so you can find in your life this creative power to make your dream come true. It could be as simple as feeling your peace and pure intentions transforming into a powerful happy feeling, or it could involve months and years of planning to see a seed idea or project become a reality.

In the East, there are many statues of Laughing Buddhas doing this Summer Chi Kung Exercise. I was surprised to see a Laughing Buddha statue in an oriental garden on the way to Plymouth, in the south-west of England. He was about 3.5 metres (12 feet) high and over a metre (4 feet) in diameter, with a huge belly and a big laughing face. Looking at such a face is like looking at the face of Mother Nature. The face of summer is a face bursting with colourful flowers of a million shades and tones. Being happy is your natural right.

Many people need rushes of adrenaline and life-risking experiences to keep them feeling high, and for them that is happiness. But when they do not have those highs, they are like drug addicts looking for their next fix. On the ground, where you are, just next to you, a little flower is dancing with the wind, an ant is climbing up a tree. You look up and there you see a bird gliding above you, a cloud very slowly moving towards you – these simple moments can be ecstatic if you slow down to feel the simple cosmic life force ebbing and flowing in them. On the one hand, you may be able to feel these kinds of ecstatic experiences in still meditation. On the other hand, you could also feel the Chi Kung and T'ai-Chi movement as a naturally ecstatic celebration.

Another way to experience this joy in action is when you have difficult and serious situations confronting you: ask yourself, 'What is the funny side to this situation?'

Let me give you an example. Recently, I was on a train journey to London from Cornwall and I had forgotten my portable cassette player. I usually use it to play relaxing music on this four-hour journey. I had a problem. How could I manifest a walkman? I asked the train barman and he suggested I ask the ticket collector. The ticket collector told me to ask the other passengers. For the first time, I realized how serious I was. I needed a walkman – and I needed it badly!

I walked up and down the train looking for someone with a walkman. When I asked one passenger whether he would like to rent it to me or to sell it to me, I found a receptive ear. We were even bargaining a bit over the price, and then it emerged that he wouldn't accept a cheque. Only cash. I did not have enough. So I thanked him and left him. Halfway back to my seat I stopped by the window between the carriages and burst out laughing at my silly predicament. Not many people would wander up and down a train asking complete strangers if they could borrow or purchase their cassette players. Before this moment, I would never have imagined I had the nerve to go around asking people if they had a walkman.

With a sense of light-heartedness I went back to my seat and began to do something else which absorbed my attention. Then I noticed that a man sitting quite near me was not using his walkman. He lent it to me free of charge!

☯ Sixth Chi Kung Exercise/Principle Autumn

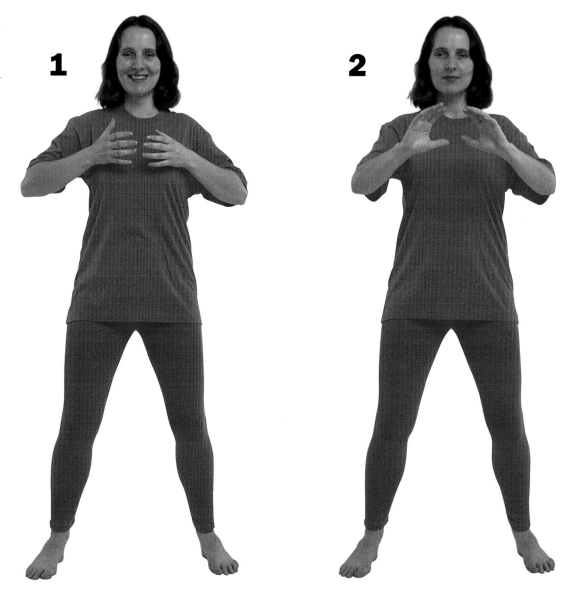

1 **2**

1–2 From the last part of the Summer Chi Kung exercise (see page 102), feel the joy of the fruit-bearing cycle of Nature change into the loving energy of sharing. With your palms forming a ball shape, turn your hands outwards, in front of your chest. Keep the thumbs and first fingers in the triangular formation.

When to practise
When you feel too much by yourself and are lonely.

Best time to practise
Any time during the day.

Tao of Orange lessons
There is a ripe time to give of yourself to others and to give with joy in your heart. As you share the fruits of your labour, the seeds of goodness take root in the people you share with. These seeds grow in their turn and continue the kindness you have sown.

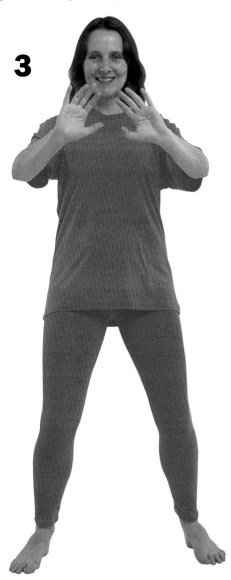

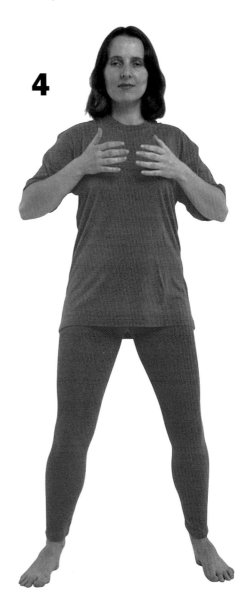

3 Push out slightly further, keeping your elbows are arched so that you create another circular shape with your bent elbows and palms.

4 Bring both palms back to your chest to form a ball of chi. Prepare for the Winter Chi Kung Exercise now.

☯ *Seventh Chi Kung Exercise/Principle*
Winter

When to practise
When you feel confused
and under a lot of pressure
and you have insufficient
emotional space.

Best time to practise
At home in the evening.

Tao of Rose Red lessons
Turn in on yourself and be
gentle and loving as you reflect,
digest and assimilate the day's
experiences.

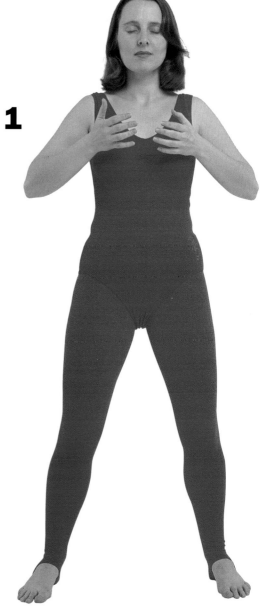

1

1–2 Starting from the final Autumn Chi Kung posture (page 107), slowly turn your palms downwards.

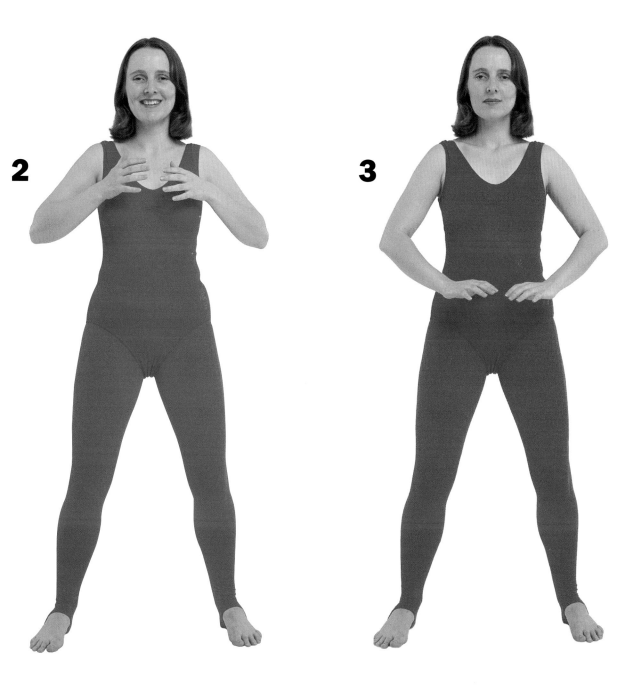

3 With your fingers and thumbs forming a triangle as before, let them sink gently down towards your tan-tien area.

Now you can begin the whole cycle of the Four Seasons again by turning your palms upwards towards your chest. Start with the Spring exercise

(see page 100), then work your way through Summer (page 102), Autumn (page 106) and Winter.

Sharing the fruits of your labour

After the Summer movement, you move into the Autumn rhythms, where you store and share your fruits with friends and relatives. The elemental powers of Nature at this time of year also demonstrate this. The gales and winds blow leftover fruits to the ground, and insects and animals distribute them throughout the land. This can be a gentle and natural way to allow people to experience the joyful abundance from you. The loving power in your hands carries the fruits of your labour with clear intentions. The fingers and thumb arrangement, symbolizing the triangle of balance of receptivity, emissiveness and creativity, is also important. Sharing is an art.

Sharing from the heart can be a balance of giving and receiving in terms of learning how to cry out not only the desire to be loved, but also the desire to give love. Creating the space to feel this powerful, loving sharing is what this movement can be about. However, Nature teaches us that we need to go through the Spring and Summer stages first. Autumn can be an ego-shattering experience. It create a feeling of emptiness and loneliness inside you, especially if the fruits of Summer plans did not come out in the positive way you hoped. Autumn can seem a dull and grey time, with rain and cold winds blowing away at you. However, there are also positive aspects to Autumn. You start to sense the beauty of the radiant colours of Autumn leaves – gold, yellow, orange and brown. You feel poetic. You feel

like singing. You feel like painting. You feel creative and alive. You feel like sharing with someone special.

Returning home to the roots of your being

After the Autumn cycle comes Winter. It is a time of returning home to yourself, to energize and conserve your energies. It is a time to hibernate and to take care of the inner fireplace (in your tan-tien centre). It is a time to rediscover that peaceful and loving place in you, to find once more a sense of wholeness through your Yin (receptive, feminine), Yang (emissive, masculine) and Tao (creative) aspects.

The Winter cycle is about returning to yourself. Taking special time to be alone with you. Doing this movement in front of a tree will allow you to feel more rooted. Picture yourself feeling your feet like the roots of the tree, sinking down into the earth and relaxing into it. When you feel negative and insecure,

do this Winter exercise and allow your palms to move all the negative energy from your heart down past your tan-tien centre and release it all into the earth. Breathe in deeply as you pull up your arms and out as you let go your arms go down. Do this for at least 15 minutes.

Another excellent way to release your negativity back into the earth is to do it literally. Write a letter to Mother Earth. Use a blank sheet of paper to share all your negative feelings. Thank Mother Earth for helping you to compost them. Be as intimate and spontaneous as you can. No one else is going to see this letter. Take as long as you need. One person who was very stressed and felt suicidal wrote nine pages and felt better. When you have finished your letter, go and dig a hole in the garden or in the forest and bury it. Thank Mother Earth again and then release all that you have written down. Let it go. Do your best not to talk or think about it again. Put your energy into creative activity.

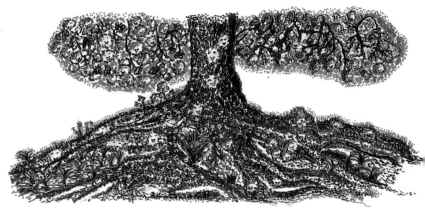

Returning home to the roots of your being

Homework 12

The Four Seasons Chi Kung Exercise/Principle

1 Practise the first three Chi Kung exercises and the Four Seasons Chi Kung Exercise every day for at least 45 minutes and record any insights you may have.

2 Describe how the Four Seasons connect to your life. If you have never thought about this before, the following questions may be helpful in giving you a start.

Generally, which areas in your life represent spring, summer, autumn and winter rhythms?

a *Spring* Do you have any 'new seed' creative projects which would bring out new feelings of enthusiasm and excitement? Think of some small steps you could take which would be the first of many steps.

b *Summer* Focusing on being in each moment, what does it mean for you to enjoy the projects? In detail (including telephone numbers, people to contact, schedule week by week, etc.) , what steps do you need to take to complete these projects? If you made mistakes in recent projects, were there moments when you could sit back and laugh about it?

c *Autumn* Do you have any plans to celebrate the completion of the seed projects you started? Have you made any 'homemade' food, created paintings, poems, stories or songs that you could share with people?

d *Winter* Which times do you find most meditative – times when you feel able to go inside to 'hibernate' and be in a contemplative mood? This is the time to write down your list of hurts and negativity and bury it into Mother Earth. This is also a time for writing to long-forgotten relatives and friends and sharing with them your peace and inspiration. Can you think of five friends with whom you would like to communicate these feelings?

Note: If any of these tasks seem too difficult, find your inner stillness again (see page 92) and listen to the waves of silence. They will bring you extra energy.

Space to record your own insights

The practice of T'ai-Chi in your daily life

Most people who have done some T'ai-Chi or Chi Kung have read about the importance of applying its principles to daily life. What frustrates them is that there are very few practical examples of how this can be done. So I hope this chapter is a small step towards remedying that.

Thousands of years ago in China, it was normal to carry a sword or flying stick with which to fight off bandits. You were looked upon with awe and respect if you knew how to use these weapons skilfully. In advanced practice of the T'ai-Chi Yielding Principle, you can apply it as a form of self-defence and learn to flow with the punches. However, our lives today are filled with stressful situations which require us to learn how to replenish our chi energy while carrying out normal activities. Students who ask me about the practice of the T'ai-Chi of the sword and the T'ai-Chi of the stick are surprised when I teach them about the T'ai-Chi of the kitchen and the T'ai-Chi of the broomstick, mop and vacuum cleaner.

You really can practise T'ai-Chi when you are doing your household chores. The end result is that you get a cleaner kitchen, more neatly chopped vegetables, a lovelier carpet and smarter clothes while you are practising T'ai-Chi.

Why practise T'ai-Chi in your daily life?

People get so bored with housework, routine jobs and other necessary chores. So what is missing? Is it not the 'enjoyment factor'?

The practice of T'ai-Chi in your daily life can bring you more joyous chi energy to revitalize these activities. You will be able to achieve more creative results. While you seem to be *spending* energy running around trying to deal with challenging situations, you could be *conserving* and *generating* chi energy in those moments.

How to fit T'ai-Chi into your daily life

Many of my students claim that they do not have time to practise every day. I ask them, 'So what do you do? Show me your movements. How do you spend your day?'

They show me physical actions of themselves waiting for a bus or the underground train; walking; lifting something heavy; washing dishes, ironing,

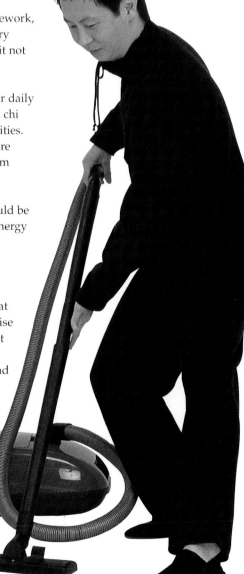

vacuuming; sitting in front of a computer, and so on. All the sorts of routine things we all do every day.

I ask them to slow down and go through the same movements with the addition of the T'ai-Chi Chi Kung principles. When they add the principle of awareness of tan-tien energy to their activities, their whole body suddenly feels much more alive and energetic. With extra energy you can accomplish more tasks with less effort. The Chi Kung principle of effortlessness in body movements means using minimal effort to produce tremendous results. The T'ai-Chi Chuan classics speak of the 'harmonious co-ordination of the lower and upper limbs from the tan-tien centre'. No matter how simple the activity you are performing is, you can still put this idea into practice.

Slowing down to flow with the pages of this book
Yes, right now, we can put the T'ai-Chi principles into practice.

First of all, slow down your actions to rediscover the awareness of what you are doing on a physical level. As you are sitting there flicking over the pages of this book, consider that even such a simple action could be a T'ai-Chi movement. Move the page very, very slowly. Be aware of your tan-tien centre moving with your elbow, wrist, palm and fingers. Be aware of your tan-tien centre not just moving 'with' your hand, but moving your whole arm.

If you do this correctly, you will feel a tingling sensation flowing through your arm and the rest of your body.

It doesn't matter which hand you use. Do it with both, one after the other. This simple movement will help generate more energy and you will feel less strain in your posture while reading.

While waiting for . . .
What about when you are waiting for a bus/train/taxi? You can practise the Eighth Fundamental T'ai-Chi Exercise (see page 76). Shift your weight from one foot to the other – again, very slowly. You are practising the T'ai-Chi principle of Substance and Non-Substance,

emptying one foot and filling up the other. This simple exercise will help you find more balance and feel more grounded. Learning to think literally on your feet may help you make wise decisions while waiting to go to your next appointment.

An exercise for learning the T'ai-Chi walking meditation
Co-ordinate your walking motion, in both your upper and lower limbs, from the tan-tien centre. There is a gentle swing from the movement of the waist. This will allow chi energy to flow through your whole body.

Be aware of the spaces between your footsteps. People who love going for walks or rambling may want to use this exercise to obtain more stamina and vitality. How do you know you are doing it correctly? If you are, you will feel the chi circulating through your feet from the earth and linking your whole body with the heavenly chi energy.

Learning to centre with breath control while lifting
Everyone has to lift heavy objects sometimes, and many people suffer from severe lower back pain because they do not know how to conserve chi energy while lifting. Often, people unconsciously contract their stomach muscles and brace themselves for the worst; then they bend over to lift the object in question. This movement pushes out oxygen, sends anxiety into the muscular and nervous system, and results in unnecessary strain.

This is what you do to correct that. Breathe in before lifting the object. Hold that breath by taking a pause. As you do this you are conserving

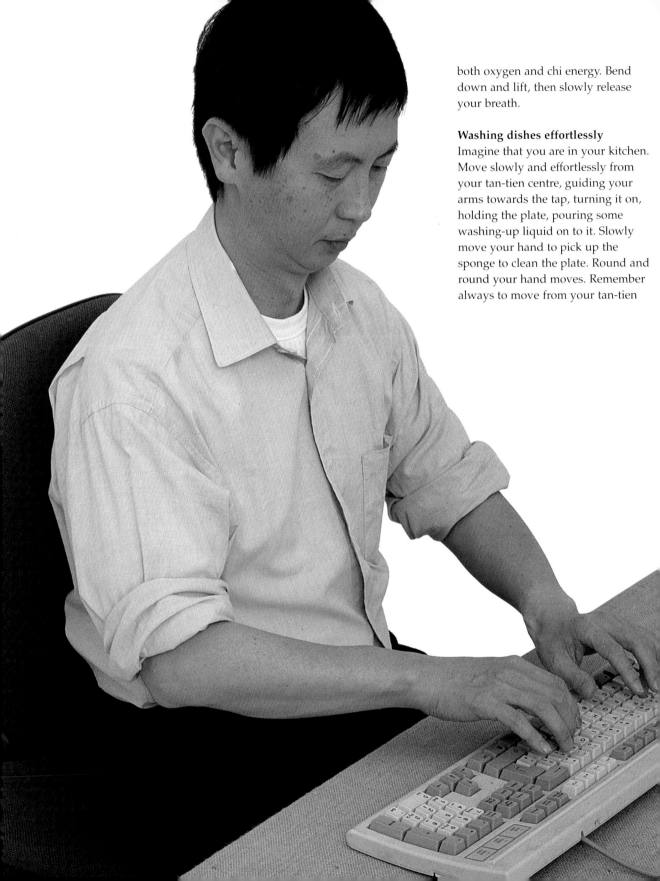

both oxygen and chi energy. Bend down and lift, then slowly release your breath.

Washing dishes effortlessly
Imagine that you are in your kitchen. Move slowly and effortlessly from your tan-tien centre, guiding your arms towards the tap, turning it on, holding the plate, pouring some washing-up liquid on to it. Slowly move your hand to pick up the sponge to clean the plate. Round and round your hand moves. Remember always to move from your tan-tien

centre. Now you will be able to use any kitchen clean-up as a T'ai-Chi meditation-in-movement exercise.

Enjoy effortless vacuuming and generate chi energy at the same time

Sometimes I bring a vacuum cleaner to my T'ai Chi Chi Kung class. Some students think they have come to the wrong course. I reassure them by demonstrating how to use the tan-tien centre to do the vacuuming. Hold the flex in one hand and the handle in the other. Taking one step forward, sink your weight into the front foot. At the same time, move your arms from your tan-tien. Pull the vacuum cleaner back effortlessly by allowing your waist to guide the arm holding the handle. When you feel a lot of chi energy, breathe it in. This is the Chi Kung breathing exercise for conserving energy. You feel as if you can vacuum the whole house when you thought that you would just do one room!

The art of ironing to smooth your chi energy

You may notice how much strain there is around your neck and shoulders when you do the ironing. And you may even find yourself using excessive effort to push the iron down and forward. Naturally you get tired and fed up about ironing. But what if you consider ironing also as a T'ai-Chi meditation-in-movement?

So, if you are ready, imagine that the ironing board is in front of you. Take one step forward, putting your foot under the board. If you are right-handed, step forward with your left foot and vice versa. Hold the iron with minimum effort and move from

your tan-tien. Do this very slowly to get the chi circulating. Place your other hand on the garment you are ironing. Co-ordinate your movements from the waist. I find my clothes feel vibrant and cosy when I iron them this way. You will discover more joy if you do all your household chores with the same attitude.

The T'ai-Chi art of mopping

One lady in a recent class shared her feelings of weariness about household chores such as mopping the floor. I asked her to demonstrate to us how she mopped and I immediately understood why she got aches and pains in her shoulders and elbows. She held the mop like a solider holding a rifle and tensed her arms in order to push it to and fro in a straight line.

According to T'ai-Chi principles, nothing in life travels in a straight line. I persuaded her to relax her elbows and shoulders. When she did this and felt a spiral-like motion of the mop moving from her tan-tien and waist, she realized that mopping could be a smooth and enjoyable activity filled with chi energy. I invite you to try it.

The T'ai-Chi Chi Kung method of painting houses

In another class, a student complained, 'I have to earn a living. I just don't have time to practise.' He had backache and lots of tension in his shoulders and neck. I asked him what he did for a living and he said he was a painter. I asked him to show me the physical dynamics of his movements while painting a house. He showed me how he held a long stick with the brush head at the end of it. He went through the

motion of moving the stick up and down the wall. His shoulders and neck were static and his arm movements were not connected to his tan-tien.

I made him slow down the movements for a few seconds. He exclaimed impatiently, 'But I can't go that slowly in my work!'

I shared with him that he needed to slow down for only about eight seconds in order to feel some benefit. I also had to be very direct with him: would he rather spend hours looking around for a good healer, osteopath or whatever to help him relax and bring him back to his natural energy? So he slowed down. I asked, 'Can you feel the chi energy now?' 'Mmm,' he said. 'Yes, yes.'

Typing using T'ai-Chi principles

Many people who spend a lot of time at a keyboard need to learn how to re-energize themselves. Aches and pains in the wrists, fingers, neck and shoulders can easily be taken care of if you slow down every 15 minutes to connect to the chi. To practise this, sit at a keyboard. It doesn't matter whether you are working at a computer, playing computer games or playing the piano. The same principles apply to all these situations. Lift your hands about 5cm (2in) up from the keys. Move your palms from your elbows, your elbows from your waist, and your waist from your tan-tien centre. Close your eyes and do this for about 30 seconds.

This simple exercise will help you to relax your shoulders, arms and spine, and give you extra energy to carry on with your work.

Your personal examples

After practising the exercises with a T'ai-Chi awareness in your daily life, you may also discover new ways to apply the T'ai-Chi principles. There is an overflowing of abundant chi energy from your tan-tien. It spills over in little actions – for example when you are seated and not doing anything in particular, can you think of how even such a simple body posture can be a T'ai-Chi movement? Write down your own personal examples in the areas of activity listed below.

In the garden

_____

_____

_____

In the shops

_____

_____

_____

In the office

_____

_____

_____

Other examples

_____

_____

_____

T'ai-Chi Chi Kung for children

The following pages outline a special programme to help children aged seven to twelve relax and discover natural harmony in their body movements. Children are naturally drawn to the movements of T'ai-Chi and Chi Kung because they are already tuned in to the chi energy. They do it unconsciously.

Some exercises are more suitable to their needs than others. So, the following exercises have been adapted from those in the earlier part of this book, and I have found them very successful in helping children to relax and to remember their inherent vital force.

Children's apparent inability to endure long hours of sustained practice of these exercises reveals that in fact they do not need it. They can connect to the chi in just 15–30 minutes.

The following explanations are designed to be read by a parent or older friend or relative. It is, of course, preferable for that older person to learn the exercises themselves before attempting to teach and guide the child to do them. The connection with natural images – such as the snow melting and the seagull flying – is a particularly effective way of helping children understand the philosophical principles behind the exercises.

First T'ai-Chi Exercise
The spider climbing and the snow melting experience

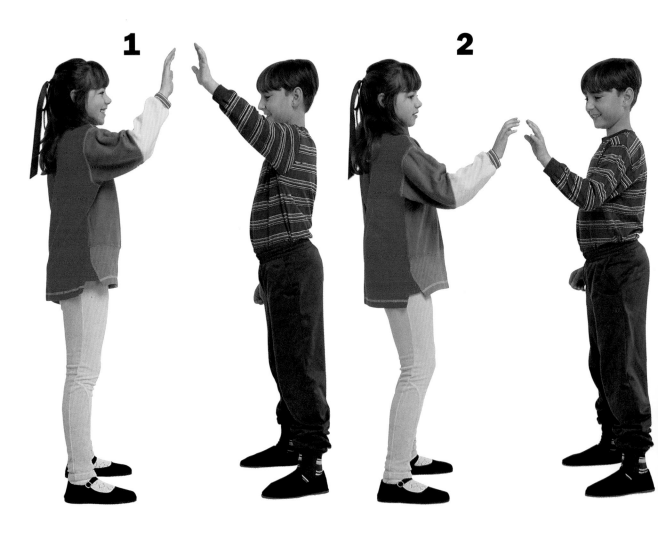

1–2 With your feet shoulder-width apart, gently swing your arm up like a spider climbing a window pane on a cold winter's day. As your fingers and palms come down slowly in a zig-zag, imagine the snow melting on the window pane, like tiny raindrops falling down. Then do the same thing with the other hand. Do this for a few minutes.

This exercise is a good starting point for indirectly introducing a child to the concept of rejuvenation without even talking about it!

Third T'ai-Chi Exercise
Embracing the tree experience

Put your right palm on your chest
and the other hand on your stomach.
Can you feel your breathing?
Breathing in, breathing out.
Breathing in, breathing out.

Breathe in again. Pause. Breathe out.
Pause. Breathe in again. Pause.
Breathe out. Pause.

Now, with your right palm, can you
feel your heart beating? Feel the
heartbeats coming into your palm.
Let your heart come to you rather
than trying to hear it. Feel it.

This exercise is one of the most
calming and peaceful for both
children and adults. You can do it
standing in the normal way, with
your feet apart, or try it sitting or
even lying down.

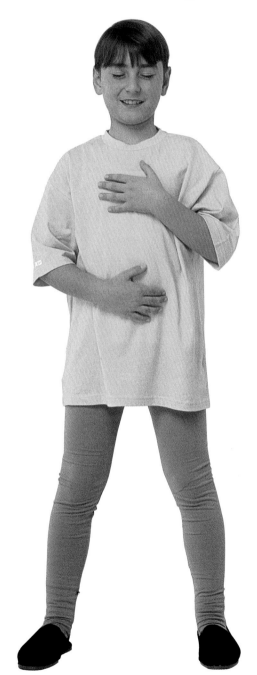

Sixth T'ai-Chi Exercise
The seagull experience

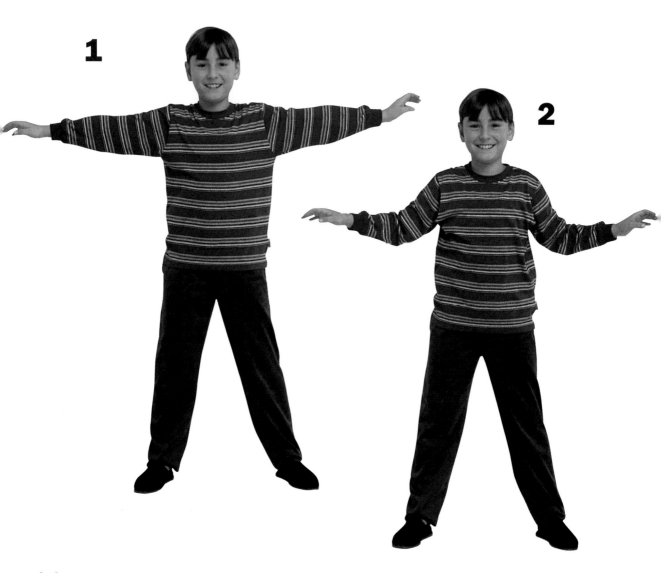

1–2 With your feet shoulder-width apart, spread your arms out slowly to your sides the way a large bird opens her wings. Imagine that you are a seagull flying, swooping down to catch fish and then gliding up again. Allowing your elbows and upper arms to move the lower arms up and down requires a conscious effort. With a gentle flick from the tan-tien, feel your arms floating in slow motion in the air. Feel them floating down in slow motion.

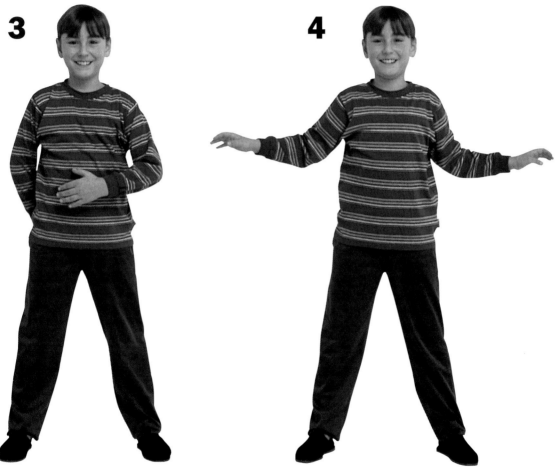

3 Place your right hand on your tan-tien centre and the other in the same position behind you.

4 Then, using your waist, gently flick your hands up again.

This exercise is energetic and dynamic and requires space for children to run around and feel their gliding arms floating freely like a bird. Some boys prefer to imagine themselves as aeroplanes, and that is okay too.

Eighth T'ai-Chi Exercise
The fountain experience

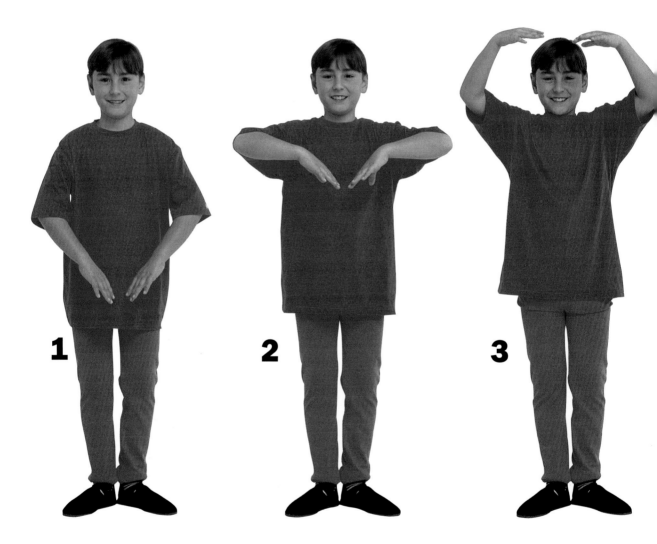

1 Stand with your heels together and your feet in a V-shape. Bring your hands together back to back and feel your arms lifting up very, very slowly.

2 Let your elbows lift your arms from above, up to shoulder height.

3 Sink your elbows down, open your arms out and extend your lower arms upwards, like a flower opening her petals.

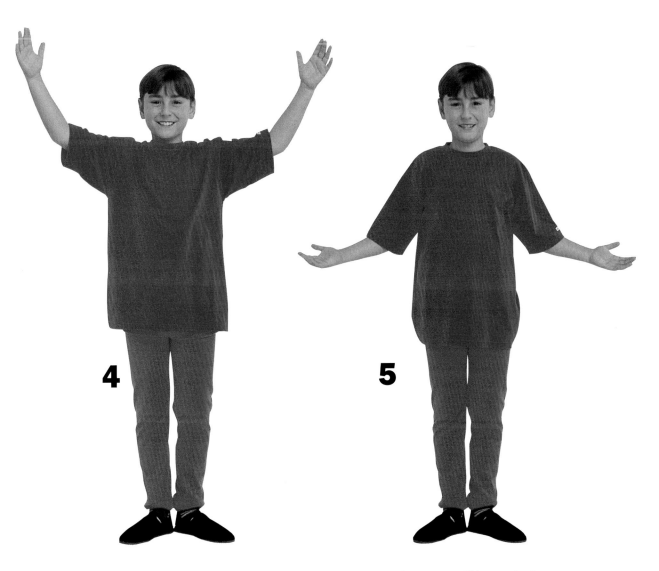

4 **5**

4–5 Feel your palms facing the sky, stretched out to your sides and floating as they fall down in slow motion.

Do this 7 times. This exercise is very beneficial for circulating the chi energy from the feet upwards through the whole body.

First Chi Kung Exercise
The tree rooting experience

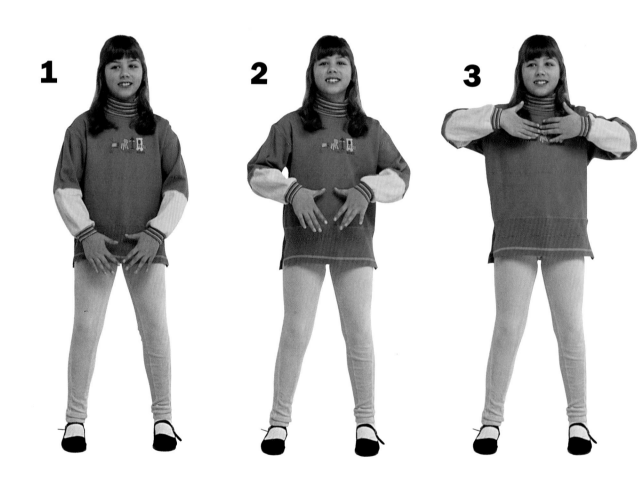

1–4 With feet shoulder-width apart, reach down with your fingers. Feel them going into the earth. Like a tree drawing up nurturing fluids from its

roots, bring your arms up, palms facing the front of your body. I usually ask children what their favourite tree is as they go through

this exercise. They say, 'Apple tree, pear tree, oak' and they focus on a tree they like. As their palms are in front of their abdomen, chest and

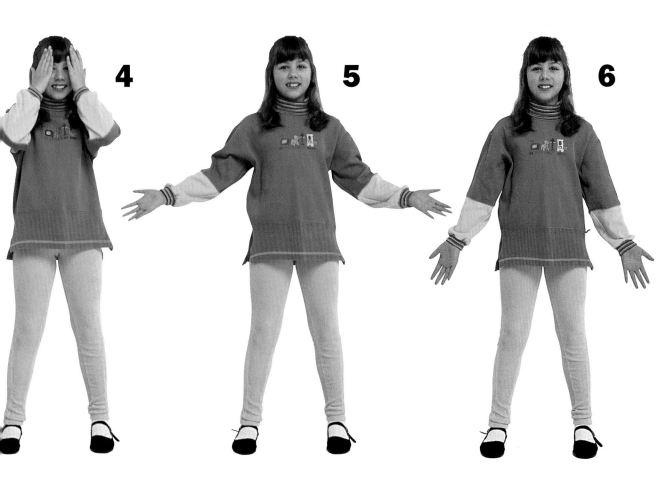

head, I add, 'You are putting lots of good energy through your palms into your stomach, kidneys, liver, spleen, heart, lungs and brain.'

5–6 Now open your palms and allow them to float down. Repeat the sequence from the ground up again.

This is a very energizing experience for the internal organs and encourages the natural harmonious circulation of chi energy in the child's body.

Second Chi Kung Exercise
The sun rising and rain falling experience

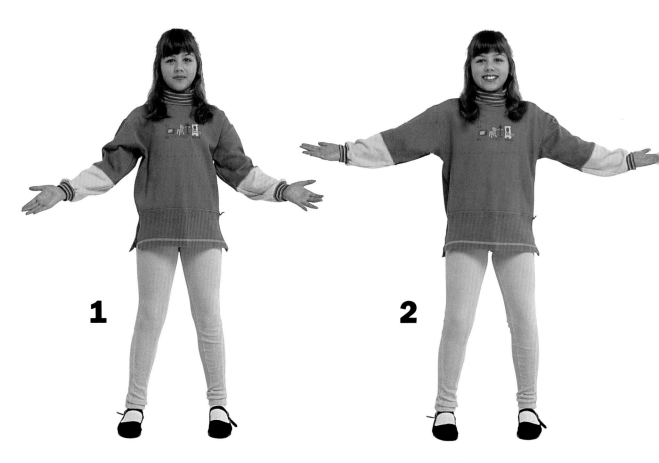

1

2

1–2 Keep your feet shoulder-width apart. With your arms at your sides, slowly open your palms so that they face the sky. Gradually, raise your palms up, up and up. You are like the sun's rays spreading outwards and upwards from the horizon into the sky. The first rays of sunlight bouncing off the tallest trees of the earth. Stretch your arms up above your head.

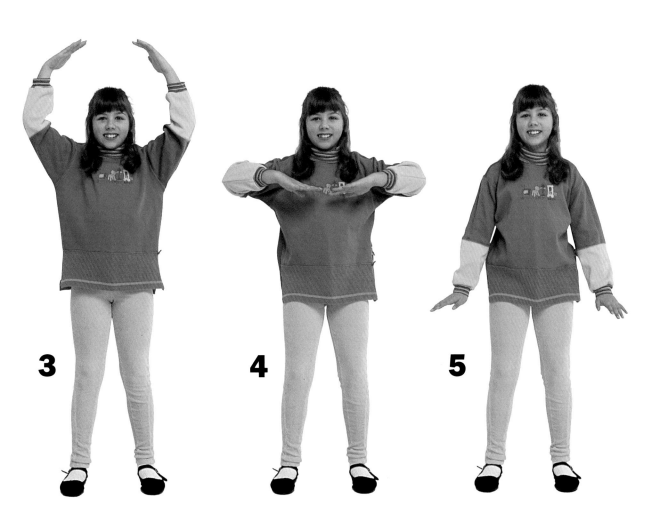

3 Then allow your hands to drop, palms facing the top of your head.

4–5 Relax your elbows and shoulders and sink your arms down, down, very slowly to the sides of the body. Like rain falling, palms in front of the midline section of your body. Sinking down and moving slowly to the sides, let your wrists bend. Pause. Then begin again.

Four Seasons Chi Kung

This exercise is based on images easily obtained from any child's experience of spring, summer, autumn and winter.

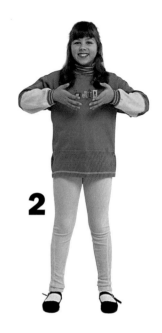

2

1–6 Draw your hands up and push out to your sides from your heart centre, like a seedling growing into

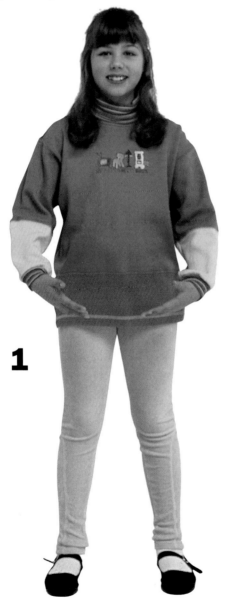

1

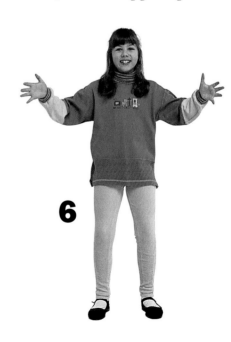

6

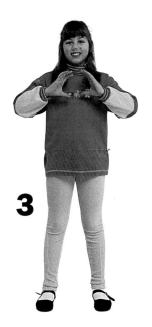

3

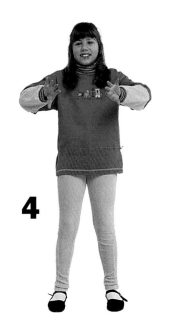

4

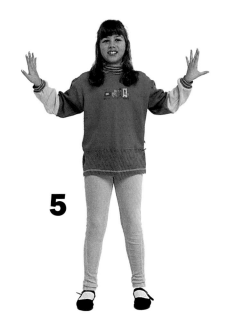

5

spring. At this point, I usually ask the child or children which flowers

grow in springtime. They often say, 'Daffodils.'

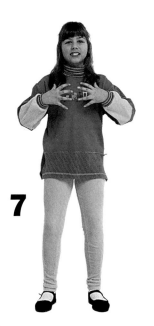

7

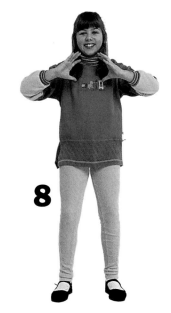

8

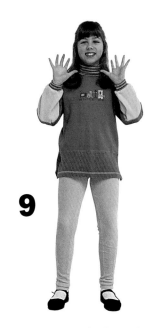

9

7–9 Bring your hands back into the heart centre and turn them round so

that the palms face your chest. (I may ask, 'What is summer like for

you? What kinds of colours do you see in Nature during summer?')

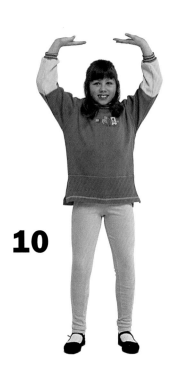

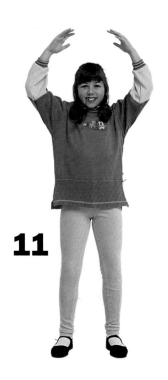

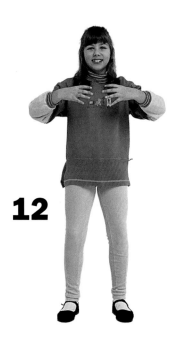

10 Push your palms up to the space above your head, holding them there for a minute.

11 Then, turn them from above your head to face the earth. Both palms sink gradually, down, down to the heart centre.

12 From the heart centre, you connect to the movement in front of the chest. (I may ask at this point, 'Now we are into the autumn season, what kinds of fruits and vegetables do you find in autumn?')

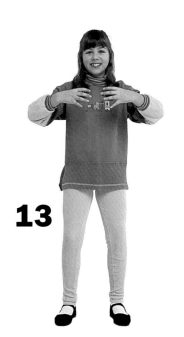

13

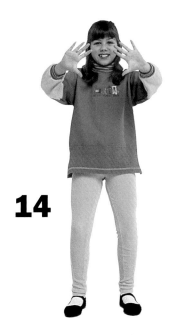

14

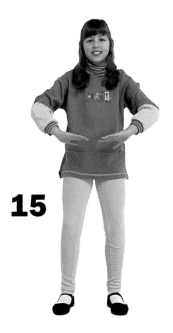

15

13 With your palms at your chest area, feel a ball of chi in between your hands.

14–15 Push forward with both palms in front of you. Pause. Bring your hands back, using your elbows to guide them towards your chest and push your palms gently down towards the earth. This is winter. We sometimes cut up different pictures

of the four seasons and, depending on the age of the children, encourage them to add their own or to put jig-saw puzzle pieces of the seasonal images together. It is also fun to go around different groups to see what kind of pictures they came up with.

The five-minute T'ai-Chi Chi Kung workout

A special programme to maintain radiant health throughout the day.

I have had occasion to train many people who live a hectic lifestyle and tell me that they are too busy to practise Rainbow T'ai-Chi Chi Kung. I take them into the exercises and they are surprised to find that they can do four exercises in less than five minutes. This is not simply going through the motions mechanically. Some people tell me that the five minutes seems much longer (five minutes can seem like five hours if you are releasing your mind into a timeless state) because their minds have slowed down to such a degree that they can feel the air thick like velvet around them. Even though you have done the exercise just once, your whole body can feel vibrant with revitalizing, tingling chi.

Do you have to be a very experienced practitioner to feel this way? Not necessarily – a beginner can be even more receptive to chi energy because of his or her humble, 'not knowing' state of consciousness. To ensure that you get maximum benefit from your daily five-minute workout, however, it is recommended that you complement it by working regularly with a qualified instructor on a one-to-one basis or attending weekly T'ai-Chi Chi Kung evening classes.

Note: For more details about the specific exercises and principles below, please refer to the appropriate sections earlier in the book.

Spring Chi Kung Exercise

(see page 100)

Time allotted
1 minute

When to do it
I would recommend you to do this exercise first, just after you get up or when you are about to leave home to go to work.

Why do it
You will achieve a stronger sense of optimism and joy around you when you take the first steps into the world.

Bring your palms to your heart and stretch them out to the sides slowly and purposefully. The Spring energy is there within you, so that you start the day with a spring of energy inside you. You are like a budding seed opening its seedling case into two halves and stretching to make way for the new to spring up.

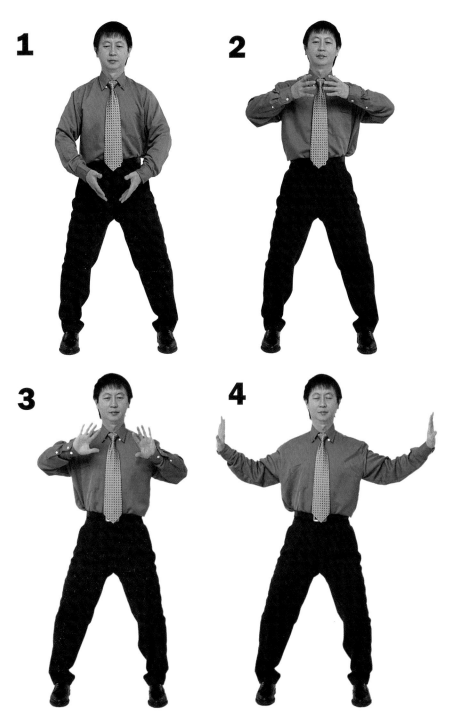

Second T'ai-Chi Exercise

(see page 30)

Time allotted
1 minute

When to do it
Around midday or whenever it gets hectic. Many people I have worked with have found this exercise helpful because it is practical and deals with the stressful situations that inevitably arise during the day. Many have also found it useful when they have to make decisions. If you feel too self-conscious to do it in the office, excuse yourself, go to the toilet and do it there. It will take less than a minute.

Why do it
This exercise will help you transform difficult decision-making issues by bringing you into a more balanced state of well-being.

Sit down and bring both hands together on your lap. Put any negative images and feelings you have into your left hand and positive images and feelings into the right. If you find it difficult to feel the positives, a simple question could bring out the right answer: 'What positive lessons am I learning/can I learn from this situation?' Bring both palms together in your heart, then let them sink down slowly to your tan-tien. Pause there for a few seconds. Feel the warmth between your palms and the tan-tien. Melt into that tingling warmth and feel revitalized.

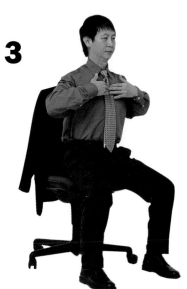

1

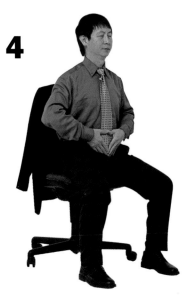

2

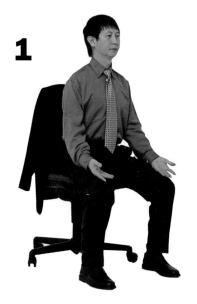

3

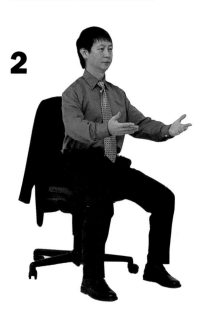

4

Third T'ai-Chi Exercise

(see page 40)

Time allotted
2 minutes

When to do it
Just before you sleep or before you get up from bed. Useful also from midday to the evening. This exercise allows you to connect calmly to your heartbeat listening and your breathing listening; it centres you. You can also add a sense of gratitude to this exercise. Being appreciative of your body's organs, your bed, your pillow, the people around you, your toothbrush, the bathroom, the house, the floor, the car, the office, etc., helps to prepare your consciousness ready for the day.

Why do it
This exercise will bring you a deep sense of peace and harmony, helping to prepare you to greet the world in a relaxed state of mind.

Lie down and place one palm on your heart (support your elbow with a small pillow if your arm feels uncomfortable) and the other palm on your belly. Concentrate on your breathing. Listen to the pauses between your in-breath and out-breath and to the pauses between your heartbeats.

First Chi Kung Exercise

(see page 86)

Time allotted
1 minute

When to do it
At the end of the day. This exercise helps you to get back in touch with your body when you have had a long day. It also energizes your internal organs after your evening meal.

Why do it
This exercise is vital if you want to live to a healthy old age. It encourages you to be kind and sensitive to your internal organs and keep them healthy and loving.

Stand with your palms and fingers in front of your thighs. Draw chi energy up your legs to cross your tan-tien and pause in front of your stomach area. Move both palms up, slowly, in front of your kidneys, then over your liver, spleen, heart and lungs. Use this exercise to energize your internal organs. As your palms reach the front of your face, let their tingling warmth relax your whole face. Then release both palms to float gently down to earth.

Physical chi healing

How to use the T'ai-Chi Chi Kung principles to accelerate natural healing

T'ai-Chi is born out of infinity. It is the origin of the positive and the negative. When T'ai-Chi is in motion, the positive and the negative separate; when T'ai-Chi stops, the positive and negative integrate.

Wong Chung-yua, T'ai-Chi Master 1600 AD

The gradual deepening of our understanding of these timeless Taoist principles opens the dimensions of chi healing. This chapter is specially dedicated to chi healers all over the world who often work behind the scenes of conflicts.

What is chi healing?

Chi healing is based on the Chinese Taoist medical philosophy. It is believed that all illnesses/stresses/pains are the result of imbalances in the body. The balancing of the Yin (receptive) principle of the soft chi energy of the healer and the Yang (emissive) principle of the patient's hard chi energy enables a harmonizing effect to take place. This state of harmony – and health – may be permanent or temporary, depending on the skills of the chi healer and the receptivity of the patient to chi energy.

What are the benefits of chi healing?

Chi healing is non-intrusive and relaxing. It involves very little physical contact. Research has found that chi energy is very effective in healing ailments caused by disorders of the nervous system, such as depression, vomiting and pains and disorders of the stomach, intestines, shoulders, lower back and heart. It can also help sports injuries such as muscular cramps, sprains and aches to heal faster in a natural way.

Chi healing helps the body to release endorphins (the body's natural painkillers) and can be used as a temporary form of pain relief – it can ease toothache while you are waiting to see a dentist, for example. It can also help to cure some illnesses in their early stages.

Research at the First Medical Academy in Shanghai, China, shows how T'ai-Chi Chi Kung practice helped patients suffering from ulcers, depression, vomiting, stomach pains, abdominal distension and nervous disorders. Chi healing can help people to feel calmer before medical operations, and it can speed the recovery process after illness or surgery. It cannot help those suffering from hereditary illnesses or viral infections.

In advanced chi healing, qualified healers can help clients with a strong chi energy level to achieve permanent healing results from the conditions listed above.

Your response to chi healing depends on how receptive you and the chi healer are to chi energy. You should not take any strong medication or strong drink such as coffee or alcohol on the day before you have a chi healing session.

You are advised to practise chi healing exercises in conjunction with other complementary health treatments and to consult your doctor before commencing any programme of chi healing or self-healing. Never stop taking medicines prescribed by your doctor without consulting him/her first.

So how does chi healing work?

Chi healing is for the whole person, with a great deal of emphasis on the heart/body/mind/spirit approach. Here are a few of the guidelines we use in our chi healing courses:

1 Heartbeat listening

In Chinese medical theory, the heart is the 'governor' of the chi energies flowing in the body. So, not only is it important to listen to the 'governor', but the 'governor' needs to be given space to listen to his or her subjects too!

Learning to feel the rhythm of your heart builds a bridge between you, the earth's rhythms, the universe's rhythms and the healer's rhythms.

Chi healers first have to practise this intensively for themselves for at least six months and integrate this heart-felt awareness in relation to their daily living.

Why is this important in chi healing?

It slows down the mind, enabling you to feel the chi energy present in your body and activate a sense of wholeness in the healing process. A client may come to a session without any specific ailment or illness. After the heart connection is made, the chi healer can sense where the healing needs to take place.

2 Tan-tien (belly) centre breathing
You increase your sense of concentration when you focus on your breathing. There are a number of different techniques of breathing. Breathing from the abdomen is an important part of the healing, so that the client can 'sink' the heart energy into the tan-tien centre. This centre is usually located about two finger-widths below the navel (see page 18 for more details of this).

Concentrating the breath and heart-awareness on the tan-tien can help centre you and conserve energy. Like a storehouse, in times of need it can offer support and help to other, less healthy parts of the body hungry for healing chi energy.

3 The healing hand is a listening palm
The alignment of the heart and belly centres leads the patient and chi healer to sense blockages at different meridian points and lines of energy in the body. Sometimes the chi healer is like a traffic policeman waving his hands to signal the traffic to move on, to free up the flow of energy and restore harmony.

To do this correctly, the chi healer has to pause and allow his or her palm to 'listen' to the body's energies speaking to him or her. The body enjoys speaking to you in different mediums. Some patients 'see' black or grey spots transform into brilliant white lights; others 'feel' different sensations such as heaviness or lightness, sharpness or smoothness and hot or cold breeze.

If there are unusually strong blockages, an effortless and gentle movement of the palm to 'pull out' the blockages can be interpreted as simply returning heavy energy to the earth. Everything that feels heavy sinks into the ground. The earth naturally transforms the 'dirty' energy into valuable compost! The end result is often a sense of freedom, ease, comfort and release from pain. All this is helping you to return effortlessly to a harmonious state of well-being.

4 Clear verbal and silent levels of communication
Such levels of communication between chi healer and client are as essential as their common focus on the chi energy as their guide. Clients and chi healers are encouraged to communicate with each other verbally at first, then gradually to flow into a deeper and deeper sense of well-being. Trusting the chi energy to be an intelligent guide is paramount to the success of every healing.

Basic preparation before a chi healing session

Before visiting a chi healer, you can do some healing work on yourself using the Fundamental T'ai-Chi exercises given earlier in this book.

For best results, you need individual assessment to establish the unique programme of exercises that is most suited to your needs, but the Second

Fundamental T'ai-Chi Exercise and Principle have been found to be most useful for many conditions causing general discomfort. On the next page you will find a shortened version of this exercise (see page 30 for the full version). This shortened version is especially useful for people who have pains in their arms

or shoulders or who cannot stand up properly. You can also do this exercise inwardly, using your emotional and mental bodies, if you are unable to do it physically – for example because of extreme illness or an accident. The chi energy provides general pain relief while you are waiting for medical help.

1

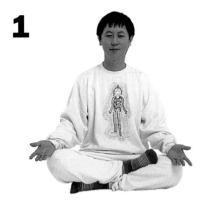

2

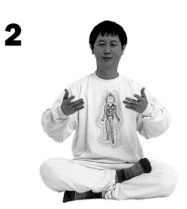

3

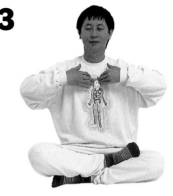

1 Sit on the floor or on a chair and concentrate on any two opposing parts of yourself. One part of you may feel pain, or may be nervous about going to see a chi healer, while another part feels that this chi healing may help you get better. You may have heard from a friend about the positive effects of chi healing, for example. Gently put the negative

self-image/feeling into your left hand and find a corresponding positive self-image/feeling to put into the right hand. You may need from 5 minutes to an hour for this stage, depending on how receptive and slow you are during and after the crisis/pain/illness. In many cases the negative can seem over-whelming, so you need to find the

positive. Ask yourself, 'What lessons can I learn from this situation? What can I appreciate about this?'

2-3 Slowly bring the two parts together. Place both palms on your chest and let them stay there for a minute. Feel your heartbeats. Feel the warm, tingling chi energy and melt into it.

4

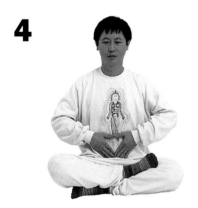

5

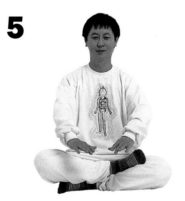

6

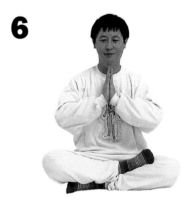

4 Sink your palms into your tan-tien, forming a triangle with your fingers, and let them stay there for 2 minutes. Feel yourself sinking into your tan-tien and remain there. Move your hands 2–3 cm (about an inch) away from your body and keep on feeling the warm, tingling chi energy. Keep melting into it. Be quiet, peaceful and in stillness.

5 Open your palms so that they face forward and place them a few centimetres (inches) away from the painful part of your body (perhaps your knees). If you cannot reach that part of your body – for example, if you are suffering from back ache – visualize it. See it between your palms. In such a case your palms are facing each other (instead of facing down as in the photo) with about

7-12 cm (3–5 in) between them. Keep your hands in that position for 15–30 minutes, gently opening and closing them. Feel the warm, tingling energy inside the injured part of your body, accelerating the natural healing processes.

6 Bring both palms together. Feel grateful for chi energy.

Some responses to chi healing

Early in 1997, as part of their training, my Advanced Foundation T'ai-Chi and Chi Kung (F3T) students were asked to do a chi healing fieldwork project in their own locality. They invited students, friends, colleagues and relatives to try chi healing and find out how it could benefit them. These 'clients' were informed that chi healing methods coul be used in co-operation with conventional medical treatments and complementary health therapies.

A total of 120 chi healing sessions were conducted. Clients filled in feedback forms after each session and a follow-up questionnaire two weeks later. We have now received 81 feedback forms and they gave us a lot of insights into the effectiveness of the chi healing experience.

The first question on the form asked the client to describe the nature of their stress/pain/illness. Some provided a detailed medical history. The majority described aches and pains in the neck, shoulders, chest, lower back and joints. A third suffered from arthritis, asthma, headaches, numbness or stiff muscles in different parts of the body caused by accidents.

The second question concerned any other forms of treatment and medication they were using. Of those who took medication, about 50 per cent used conventional forms of treatment, such as pain-killers, prescribed by doctors. The other half used herbal and alternative methods to work on their problems before coming to the session.

The third question was, 'What effect did the chi healing have on your stress/pain/illness? Ninety-five per cent of the answers mentioned feelings of relaxation, freedom from the pain/stress/illness, and calmness. Clients also used expressions such as 'I feel tingling warmth' and 'I was aware of a rippling energy' when they reflected on the impact of the chi healing on specific parts of their bodies.

Clients were also asked how they felt after the chi healing session. Ninety per cent felt more centred, peaceful, happier and said that their pain/stress/illness either improved dramatically or disappeared completely. Those who suffered from stress and physical pains reported a total recovery. Others, who complained of a wide variety of problems, including hypertension, angina, osteoporosis, blocked energy in the solar plexus, irritable bowel syndrome, high blood pressure, inflammation of muscles, exhaustion, sciatica and shingles, reported increased self-confidence, improvement in health and a general sense of well-being.

Clients were also asked to award marks out of ten for the chi healer's ability to assess their situation. The average score of 9.2 was a pleasing reflection of the healers' high degree of receptivity.

So what conclusions can we draw from this feedback? Firstly, people who had been practising their T'ai-Chi and Chi Kung exercises regularly before and/or after the sessions were able to achieve more satisfactory healing results than those who did not. They were better able to tune in to the chi healing frequency and initiated their own self-healing processes. Many of these people also underwent other health treatments and practices which were complementary to their T'ai-Chi and Chi Kung sessions, such as the Alexander technique, aromatherapy, homoeopathy, reflexology, osteopathy, acupuncture, meditation, and yoga.

On the other hand, there were some clients who did not believe in chi healing or any kind of complementary therapy. Despite their scepticism, even some of these people were able to remark at the end, 'Hey, it works!' This category included people suffering from headaches, neck pains, shingles, back ache, muscular strains and numbness. They found relief after the chi healing sessions.

Some of the healing effects lasted only a few hours or a few days. But this happened exclusively with people who went back to stressful lifestyles and unsupportive familiar environments.

I believe, however, that some seeds have been sown and may sprout at the ripe time. The gift of a chi healing experience is that both healer and patient benefit. As the patient experiences the healing energy pulsating through him or her, so does the chi healer. These experiences remind us that the inner dimensions of healing harmony really exist and are accessible to all of us when we slow down to find our way back home and have another taste of energizing health, harmony and peace.

The following are edited accounts of the healing experiences these clients shared. I am grateful to these people for permission to relate their stories.

The first is by Andy Mcphersen of Cornwall.

For many years it had been my dream to swim with dolphins, and in October 1996 I had a fantastic experience off the beach near my home. I had paddled out on my surf-board to watch a school of dolphins playing in the waves. They were jumping clear of the water, playing and splashing their tails and riding the waves past me. I sat on my board marvelling at this spectacular and enlightening sight. Then I realized I was being dragged towards the rocks by the rip current. I wrenched my shoulder making the extra effort to paddle myself to safety. It was very painful and I felt quite panicky.

At that moment one of the dolphins surfaced just in front of me and looked me straight in the eyes. I knew that it was checking to see if I was all right. It stayed there until I was clear of the rocks, then carried on playing.

The next day I couldn't lift my arm at all, my shoulder was so painful. By coincidence I was due to see Annie Fitzgerald [one of the F3T students] for a chi healing session, and the day after that, thanks to her, I was back surfing again.

For some time I had been suffering extreme pain in my kidneys and bladder. After a couple of years of misdiagnosis, I found I had a kidney stone. After I started seeing Annie, the pain subsided. When I went to see the specialist, I was informed that the stone had moved into my bladder. By this time, my whole life felt as if it had been turned upside down. I had a virtually constant burning pain in my penis. I was stressed out at work. My girlfriend had left me and I was broken-hearted. I often woke up crying; I cried all day and cried myself to sleep. Life felt pointless and I spent one night close to suicide.

I spoke to Choy and he talked me through some exercises over the phone. Gradually I began to practise T'ai-Chi and meditate again. It was my only hope, to be with all those different aspects of myself that were crying out for attention and that I had ignored for so long.

I saw Annie regularly for chi healings and I focused on healing myself, too. Meanwhile he specialist at the hospital told me that the kidney stone was too big to pass and that I would have to have an operation which involved poking an implement up my penis, grabbing the stone, crushing it and then flushing out the pieces! I was terrified.

One of the things that Choy had suggested was that I meditate on the dolphin that had come up and looked me in the eye. I had been doing this nearly every day and I had found it incredibly moving and healing. I felt that the dolphin was still there for me and it put me back in touch with universal feelings of softness and compassion. I felt grateful for the love and I even started to like myself again. I felt that I had been giving myself a very hard time.

One evening when I was practising Rainbow T'ai-Chi Chi Kung, I had an amazing experience during the Chi Kung Kidney Exercise. I felt very connected to my kidneys. I visualized a heavy black substance being released from my kidney and imagined my kidney bright and radiant. Then the kidney transformed into a dolphin. I normally find it difficult to slow my mind down in order to visualize, yet all this happened effortlessly.

The next day I was struggling to urinate. It was taking longer and longer to do this as I felt more and more blocked by the stone. Then suddenly the stone shot out into the toilet. I was so overjoyed and excited that I burst into tears and went dancing round the house. It was an amazing experience. To pass a stone the size of a pea, with no pain!

The first thing I did was to phone Annie and she was overjoyed. She had given me a healing session the day before and said that she hadn't given up hope – she said that she had made a strong connection with my kidneys and told them that they still had time to release the stone. This was just a few days before I was due to go in for the operation!

I feel as though I have been to hell and back over the last three months, but I am so grateful for what I have learned. I have healed myself physically and emotionally. My whole life has changed. I feel more centred. I feel confident and alive. I appreciate my body. I feel joyous.

This next story is by Joy Blowes of Cleveland:
I heard about chi healing from David Baines [a T'ai-Chi instructor, FTT graduate and F3T trainee]. I was suffering from low energy and a lack of confidence, as well as creaking and painful knees and thumb. The doctor had described these pains as 'wear and tear'. I did not take medication but had been trying to improve my diet, taking cod liver oil and doing a little gentle walking instead of more violent exercise. When I started going to see David I had been having these painful symptoms for over a year.

The last two healing sessions were quite dramatic. My feet involuntarily turned inwards until the toes touched and I recalled falling off an outbuilding as a child, hurting my feet and having to wear special heels on my shoes for a while. It had happened many years ago, but I was moved to tears when I remembered it. After this session, my knee felt better and I was relaxed and happy.

At the final session I again experienced an involuntary movement: this time my thumb moved on its own across the palm of my hand. A pain then travelled up from my thumb through my shoulder. Again I felt relaxed and happy at the end of the session.

In general after these healing sessions I have more energy, more optimism and am more able to get on with the things I want to do. My knees are better and the swelling on my thumb has gone. I found chi healing powerful and beneficial. I would certainly use it again.

Carol Timms of Cornwall:
Two years ago, I began attending weekly Rainbow T'ai-Chi classes. It was my first experience of heart-centred T'ai-Chi in a supportive group where there was an opportunity to express feelings and be heard. We blended this with beautiful fluid movement – moving meditation! T'ai-Chi became something my body wanted to do, rather than something I felt I *should* do. I was inspired to practise every day, usually out of doors, by the sea or in favourite places in fields or among trees.

I began to perceive that I had been neglecting myself. In fact there was a huge amount of guilt, fear and anger from the past that I had been avoiding looking at – I had been too busy 'giving' to others. Rainbow T'ai-Chi has helped me to own, to transform and to integrate my negative as well as my positive aspects.

When I first came to Jeanne [another FTT graduate and F3T trainee] for chi healing, I had given up smoking some months before and my lungs were so badly congested that I was unable to sing without wheezing and gasping for breath. At the end of the session, we connected with a freeing, healing sound together and I came away feeling energized. I am very grateful to Jeanne and to rainbow T'ai-Chi for helping me to take responsibility for my life and for my healing. What a gift!

Joyce Rusk of Cleveland:
A childhood injury has caused me increasing back pain over the last twenty-eight years. I have a curvature of the spine and in recent years my spine has started to rotate. Pain ranges from slight aches to barely able to move and affects my whole body.

Over the years I have tried all kinds of pills, potions and remedies, including hanging upside down on an ironing board! I have been going to an osteopath for seven years and do daily stretching exercises. It was my osteopath who gave me a phone number and said, 'Try Rainbow T'ai-Chi Chi Kung.' I have been going to T'ai-Chi Chi Kung classes with David Baines for three years.

I decided to try chi healing with David because I have felt so much better about myself since I started classes. During the first healing session I felt heat going deep into my shoulder muscle, my arm felt heavy and stiff, then this was replaced by tingling in my fingers which worked its way into my hand, up my arm into my elbow.

Over the next two weeks I kept feeling the heat return. During the next session I could feel heat again and I could see flames dancing. I also felt such joy I laughed out loud!

Then one day when I was stretching my back clicked and the pain has since ceased. I know I have a long way to go yet, but there is a light at the end of the tunnel that was once dark and there is now a light in me. The deep relaxation and sense of well-being that chi healing can give must surely have a role to play in this modern stressed world.

The Tao of Rainbow T'ai-Chi Chi Kung

How to make friends with your inner self and money

This chapter is based on the Tao of Rainbow T'ai-Chi Prosperity Workshops designed for students attending classes on the fundamental T'ai-Chi Chi Kung exercises and principles.

My experience of what money is

When I was in my teens and early twenties, I worked variously as an office equipment salesman, book sales assistant, restaurant and catering manager, school teacher, copywriter, research manager, chrome factory sales executive, Chinese medical sales representative and account executive. I was also very interested in the philosophical aspects of my daily life and spent most of my spare time learning about Taoist principles, under the guidance of my father, who was a part-time Chinese medical doctor.

At work, my observation that people generally had a recognitive relationship with money was confirmed. However, I had a different perspective when my father brought wise men home: I was inspired to realize that there was a cognitive way to perceive money. A wise teacher demonstrated to us that there was a clear, harmonious link between the Yin/Yang/Tao principles, chi energy and paper money. Just as balance was essential to our physical, mental and emotional health, so failure to respect this balanced relationship would result in poverty and ill health.

A Yang attitude towards money

On a mental level, we recognize that the purpose of money is to facilitate trading in goods and services We can see how a certain sum of money can be more or less valuable 'in real terms' depending on the state of the human-created economy.

Twenty years ago, we could buy a loaf of bread for a lot less than what we pay for it now. On the other hand, a coin collector might pay hundreds or even thousands of pounds or dollars for an old coin, and suddenly something that you might have been tempted to throwinto the dustbin is worth a fortune! These relative values are something we humans have projected on to money.

Money can also be used as a means to do good for others. You can pass positive feelings into money and allow it to circulate in a beneficial way. But however good your motives may be, you still have basically a Yang attitude towards money, meaning that you recognize it as a means to achieve an end.

It is like a stranger befriending you and persuading you to do something for him: he doesn't know and does not really care who you are. This assertive or domineering attitude in the relationship with money does have consequences.

A Yin attitude towards money

So what is a receptive/Yin way of perceiving money? Fresh from school, I believed only theoretically that there was a Yin/receptive way of perceiving money. This would mean finding a receptive understanding of money as a mirror for our state of consciousness. It would mean perceiving *directly* (to cognize) what money is and allow 'money' to share with us what it is. This theory was yet to be tested.

However, such a theory was going to be put to the test at a time in my life when I least expected it. I was sitting in a bus one day, quite relaxed and in a receptive/Yin state. Suddenly, without any warning, I felt strong feelings coming from the money I had in my hand. I felt that the coins and paper money I was holding were not merely coins and paper, but substances which contained the feelings and thoughts of everyone who had handled them. At that moment, I felt overwhelmed by feelings of sadness and started crying for no obvious reason.

It took me some days before I realized that I was being the emotions in the money. During this time, I did not tell anyone about this experience with anyone in case they thought I was mad. Then I told my father and he shared with me some psychic experiences of his own that he had not told anyone either. He too had experienced spirits of material objects appearing before him regularly.

Knowing this made me feel that I was not the only one experiencing the spirit of money. However, I also wanted to understand clearly and logically what these inner experiences were all about. So I did some thinking and reading for myself.

In modern research, using Kirlian photography, scientists are discovering that there are fields of energies not only around objects which we recognize as being alive, but also around so-called non-living things. It is possible to envisage that our emotions are not only carried by objects but that emotions can be registered in the objects itself. This led me to believe that money was indeed a vehicle of human emotions.

I was not on any kind of hallucinogenic drug and I felt quite normal! But my practice of T'ai-Chi Chi Kung had slowed my mind and feelings to such a rate that I could sense the emotions in the money.

The Yin/Yang and Tao way of perceiving money

After that experience I was curious about other money that I had. I went to the bank and changed my money into notes and coins of various denominations. I tried foreign currencies, and I experienced similar feelings. It was like being introduced to a new world of 'money beings'.

I soon realized that not only could I tell what the money felt like, but I also had the choice of what kind of feelings I channelled into money. I could feel a 'sad' money being was looking for a 'happy' feeling. In this case, I would put a 'smile' into the money and found it felt better in my hand. I realized that money was also mirroring to me the sadness in my life. When I went into the Third Fundamental T'ai-Chi Exercise/ Principle (see page 40) to bring compassionate feelings into my heart and belly centre, I felt comforted and healed. I could be in a Yin/receptive/ listening state and be with what money taught me about myself. After that I could be in a more Yang/ assertive state and could verbally affirm positive feelings about money.

The Second Fundamental T'ai-Chi Exercise/Principle (see page 30) is also very useful in learning how to accept the Yin/negative and Yang/ positive aspects of our relationship with money. When, years later, I started teaching prosperity workshops, we drew Tao of Rainbow colour charts based on the Seventh and Eighth Fundamental T'ai-Chi Principles (see pages 70 and 76). These had pictures of bright, colourful energies surrounding the paper money and coins. Sometimes I would copy them on to thicker paper so that we could draw and sketch colourful vibrations around them.

As I explored all this further, I realized how unaware we could be of the fact that we had taken raw materials from Mother Nature to make all that paper money, all those coins, credit cards and cheques. I was humbled by this thought and felt immense gratitude to Mother Nature. I now saw clearly how I as a modern man could find a way back to Mother Nature by showing respect in the way I used her resources. This grateful attitude helps to strengthen our relationship with money.

Step-by-step guide to prosperity

1 Getting to know your negative beliefs and discovering your positive beliefs about money
Firstly, we need to recognize many of the projected beliefs we have put on money. Putting into practice the First Fundamental T'ai-Chi Principle (see page 26), we can let go of beliefs such as that money is the root of all evil or that having lots of

money is a good thing. The Third Fundamental T'ai-Chi Principle (see page 40) is about sensing money as it is.

Secondly, when we let go of our projections about money, we begin to realize that money is a mirror of our relationship with ourselves. If we feel insecure about ourselves, we

feel insecure about our financial situation. Feeling insecure about our financial situation is a reflection of feeling insecure about ourselves. We may start believing that money can provide the answer not just to our financial needs, but to our general insecurity. We need to see clearly that money cannot give us what we need to give to ourselves.

So, here is some homework to do. Sit down with some money in your hands. Close your eyes. Feel the pauses between your heartbeats and breathing. When you feel calm and still, ask yourself, 'What does money mean to me? What beliefs do I have about money?' Write down any negative beliefs and experiences you have about money.

An example of a negative belief might be, 'I will never be able to get that (amount of money) I need for (whatever that perceived need is).' This belief may mirror the fact that you do not feel worthy to receive help from life. Another could be, 'I envy others who have money and I hate them because . . . ' This may mirror your lack of self-esteem about the inspiring and enriching aspects of yourself which are working very hard at being creative (but perhaps not making a lot of money at it). You are not giving that part sufficient support and appreciation.

To balance the Yin and Yang aspects within ourselves (using the Second Fundamental T'ai-Chi Exercise/ Principle – see page 30), we need to discover the corresponding positive beliefs about money. You can come up with your own, or use examples such as 'All my needs are being met now. Thank you, Mother Nature. I am open to receive help from life now.' Or ' I open myself up to appreciate the homes of all rich people. As I walk past them, I can give thanks that their lovely homes give me so much enjoyment. What fine architecture. What beautiful gardens.'

So, for all the negative beliefs you have written down about money, find a corresponding positive belief. After

you have done this, go through the First and Second Fundamental T'ai-Chi exercises (see pages 26 and 30).

2 Visually build a prosperous and caring relationship with money
Continuing from Step 1, the purpose of this exercise is to create a friendlier relationship between you and a positive image of yourself. You need to give yourself at least an hour to do this exercise.

Go through the First and Second Fundamental T'ai-Chi exercises again and let go of all negative images you can recall of how you feel about money. Sit in front of a full-length mirror. Take your money out (include various denominations of notes and coins, credit card(s), cheque book(s), etc.) and place it in front of you, between you and the mirror. Spend a few minutes looking at the money and look at yourself. If you find yourself looking at those worried or tired lines around your eyes, refocus your attention. Look more closely into your eyes and see a sparkling light being vibrant with chi energy shining in your heart.

Stand up and look at your whole body. Let go of any judgmental comments about any part of it.

Close your eyes and reflect feelings of gratitude to the trees and the earth for the gift of money. Feel billions of messages of 'Thank you' pouring out to them. Feel it with all your heart, belly and mind. Feel an inner smile of gratitude shining at the earth and trees as you thank them. Feel the feelings of gratitude spreading to all parts of the earth and trees all over the planet. Spend a few minutes meditating on this.

Open your eyes and touch every piece of money in front of you with radiant chi energy. Then, look again in the mirror. What do you see now? Do you see a smiling face?

Now, using a pencil and an A4 drawing pad, sketch your prosperous, smiling and grateful face and draw only the outline of the rest of your body. Leave about a 6 cm (2½ in) space around the edges of your sketch.

Concentrate mainly on your face for the time being. You need to spend some time to get to know your face. Don't worry if you have never drawn a face before in your life. Draw an oval outline to represent your face, then an outline of the rest of your body to go with the face. Then concentrate on one area at a time, putting in your ears, nose, mouth, chin and eyes.

The first few attempts may not look much like you. Keep at it. Let go of the idea that you need to draw a perfect picture of yourself. If feelings of self-criticism persist, stop drawing and close your eyes to see which aspect of you is criticizing you. What is the motive of this 'self' who is criticizing you? If it is coming from a place of care and concern, thank the self. But if it is out to destroy your self-confidence, use the First Fundamental T'ai-Chi Exercise/ Principle to let go of the criticism and carry on your drawing.

Start a garden if you have not already done so. If your self-critical aspects are still as persistent as ever, write down their comments on a piece of paper and put the paper into the compost bin in your garden.

At the top of your drawing I would like you to write with a green felt pen, 'I am a prosperous being!' In the next few pages you will be guided to add more features to this drawing. Leave it for now and go on to the next step.

3 Acknowledging and accepting the support of the Yin/Yang and Tao aspects of you
In this step you will be using the Third Fundamental T'ai-Chi, Fifth Fundamental T'ai-Chi and First Chi Kung exercises/principles to embrace and accept the support of the Yin, Yang and Tao aspects in your whole being. This section is a continuation of your drawing in Step 2.

a Awaken your Yin/feminine/mother aspect to help you get what you want
First of all go through the Third Fundamental T'ai-Chi exercise/ principle (see page 40) to calm your mind into a state of stillness. Use your heartbeat listening and belly breathing to feel out what it is you want.

After that, sit down with your drawing and draw a loving, radiant face in the centre of your heart area. Write down the names of friends and relatives who help you to get what you want. They might or might not express this through verbal advice or gifts or whatever. Their help may take the form of emotional and/or moral support. Put their names in the heart area of your picture. You could combine this part of the exercise with the dotted lines for the feminine/ motherlike qualities. This is your Yin/feminine aspect.

I would also like you to connect to your feminine and motherlike qualities such as gentleness, tenderness, kindness, generosity,

patience, compassion and so on. It may help to think of someone in your life with whom you have experienced some of these qualities. It could be a man or a woman. Next, using coloured pens, insert these qualities as radiant dotted lines around the heart area of your drawing. Choose the colours that represent these feelings for you. One excellent way to know which colour to choose is to think of something from Nature that embodies the qualities you are trying to convey.

b Your inner Yang/masculine/father aspect can help you to go all out to get what you want
Concentrate on your breathing again. Feel the calmness increasing as you pay attention to the pauses between your in-breath and your out-breath. Be in the pauses and feel yourself melting into the stillness. Now, go through the Fifth Fundamental T'ai-Chi exercise (see page 58). Do it slowly for 5–10 minutes.

Now, sit down and draw a peaceful, smiling face in between the eyes of your face in the drawing.

Write down what you want to manifest for your life. Is it money? Put the specific amount or draw the object you want on the top of your head in the drawing. If it is a car, for example, you might have a picture from a newspaper or magazine showing what it looks like. Stick it there on top of your head. Then, in the top right-hand corner of the page, write in small letters just a few words to describe what you want to spend the money on. It could be a certain type of car. Do a bit of research in car magazines to determine exactly what you want. You might write down the

year, colour, mileage, condition of the car and the approximate cost. This is your Yang/masculine aspect.

This next part of the exercise will focus on the support of your inner father to help you go one hundred per cent to get what you want. Write the names of friends and relatives whom you feel have provided that masculine/fatherly support for you. It could be appear as a brotherly relationship you have with a friend or relative. Write down the qualities they represent for you. These may be qualities like clarity, understanding, peacefulness, confidence, persistency, hard-workingness, self-control, strength, courage and so on. Put their names and qualities at the top of your drawing, above your head, in colourful dotted lines.

Note: If you have difficulty recalling people who have expressed these feminine and masculine qualities in your life, you may be too young for this exercise to be beneficial, or you may have been very hurt and do not yet feel it is the ripe time for you to open yourself to learn to trust. This means that you need to do more practice in the Second and Third Fundamental T'ai-Chi exercises and principles (see pages 30 and 40) to rediscover more balance in yourself. There may also be some other reason why you are not yet ready to do this inner work and you may want to come back to it an another, more appropriate time.

c. Making friends with the creative spark within you
Let us continue with our example of manifesting a car. You should at this point visit a car showroom and ask for a test drive of your chosen vehicle.

This brings you one step closer to being able to affirm physically, emotionally and mentally that you already have such a car. The creative/ visual (Tao) faculty in your brain receives support from your intuitive (Yin) and rational (Yang) aspects and attitudes to universal chi energy in order to manifest what you want.

You can experiment with this creative/ visual Tao principle co-ordination with your intuitive/feeling Yin principle and logical/verbal Yang principle by applying it to simple little manifestations. I believe some people have already discovered this combination in their own daily life.

For example, recently I was in a public toilet. Just as I was feeling quite good about meditating on sending chi energy to my bowels, two men came in. One of them went into the cabin next to mine and started grunting. His friend yelled from outside, 'You know what I usually do? I imagine I have already done it!' Then I heard 'Plopp-ppp, plop, plop . . .' just beside me and a voice said, 'Yeah, it works. Thanks.' A moment later, the flushing sound and the two wise friends left the toilet. You can imagine how quiet and amused I was during this time. I am constantly amazed at how the universe keeps teaching me, even in public toilets!

Now, coming back to your car. Every day, keep visualizing that you already have the car, that you are driving it. Do this after you have practised your T'ai-Chi Chi Kung exercises, when you are relaxed. Feel that you are doing the best you can. Verbally affirm that you have this car now! Go through the First Chi Kung Exercise (see page 86), and pause

especially around your tan-tien/belly area. Feel the tingling chi around your belly. Then gently move up towards your heart to feel warm, tingling energy around your chest. You are connecting the chi to your Yin/feminine aspect. Stay there for a few minutes. Then move up to your face. Feel the tingling warmth melting any tensions around your face and feel chi energizing your Yang/ masculine aspect.

Now, sit down with your drawing and draw a smiling face in your tan-tien. Write down the names of people in your life whom you consider to be fun-loving, witty, comical, creative. Think also of wise teachers, artistic performers you like and again show them as dotted lines radiating out from the centre of that smiling face.

The creative, joyous spark within you is the result of the blending of the inner father and inner mother qualities, the dance of the clarifying/ freeing/peaceful masculine principle with the yielding/merciful/ courageous and patient feminine principle. Then comes your Tao/ creative aspect. Your source of creative inspiration could be wise teachers – if so, write their names at the top of your drawing. Above these names put a small sketch of whatever you want – a house, a car, etc.

So, now you have the Yin/feminine, Yang/masculine and Tao/creative principles supporting you in achieving what you want. You already have what you want now!

d The Tao of Colour Science
The Tao of Colour Science is based on wisdom passed down from ancient teachers of China who shared the

same belief in the power of colours as the ancient teachers of Greece, India and Egypt. They studied Nature's harmonious and wise ways of using the qualities and tones of the feminine/yin, masculine/yang and creative/Tao aspects of colour.

Most people have personal preferences for the colours of their clothes, cars, carpets, curtains, bathroom tiles, etc. Generally speaking, you may also notice that men prefer duller and darker colours and women are attracted to brighter and lighter colours. Many assistants in fashionable clothes outlets agree with me that there is insufficient choice of colours for men's clothes in comparison with women's.
It may interest you also to watch what kind of colours to which you feel attracted when you are in a certain mood. If you feel depressed, what colours do you wear? What about when you feel cheerful? In this step, I would like you to focus on how to use the Tao of Colour Science to 'clothe' events with the qualities and colours you want to manifest.

Here are some general qualitative connections with colours which I have found useful. You may like to use this as a guide for putting colourful dotted lines on your drawing.

Violet – healing, calming, forgiving
Indigo – contemplative, deep, understanding
Blue – freeing, clarifying, peaceful
Green – prosperous, harmonizing, balanced
Yellow – humble, wise, patient
Orange – happy, revitalizing, rejuvenating
Rose red – encouraging, enthusiastic, loving

4 Allow the chi energy to circulate throughout your whole house
Go through the Fourth Fundamental T'ai-Chi Exercise/Principle (see page 50) and the Kidney Chi Kung Exercise/Principle (see page 94) in whichever room you feel is the 'heart' of your house. Feel your belly centre and heart radiating chi energy and gratitude through your whole house. Move into other rooms and do the same exercises there. If a room is too small for you to do the movements, sit down and visualize yourself doing them. Play music which includes natural sounds such as dolphins, birds or water. This will help you energize the rooms faster. Round-leafed plants have been found helpful in transforming negative vibrations in a house. Try placing them in strategic corners facing the doorway.

All these aids are enabling the chi energies in your house to circulate in harmony with the universe. Some people have found it helpful to do this while standing still or sitting in a meditative posture. However, the dynamic, circular movements of the T'ai-Chi Chi Kung exercises resonate better with the way Nature flows. Nothing in Nature stays jagged for long – everything needs to curve, to bend; scientists even agree that light bends. So your house can be vibrating with energies of whatever qualities you want. Just as you choose the colour of your wallpaper or carpet, so you can choose which inner qualities you want to create in every room.

Say you want your living room to be a combination of peaceful and loving qualities – draw a colour-science picture of your room being filled with peaceful and loving blues and red. Don't forget the smiling faces!

One of my students not only did colour charts of her rooms, she decided to experiment with the walls, too. She painted the walls of her kitchen violet – the healing, calming, forgiving colour. She soon found out that this was not exactly the right colour because people started yawning, feeling sleepy and too relaxed. So, have fun but, to be on the safe side, try the colours out on paper first. When you have found the right colours and qualities, you will know by the effect they have on you and on those who visit your home.

This colour awareness is especially important when you come home after a hard day. If you have got it right, the colour and qualitative energy in your house will immediately make you feel welcome and nurtured. The house can be a sanctuary for your tired soul. It can uplift you. Inspire you. Make you feel on top of the world.

5 Acknowledging the prosperous being in you with your inner mother/father and child principles
Go through the Eighth Fundamental T'ai-Chi Exercise (see page 76) and the Four Seasons Chi Kung Exercise (page 100) to claim this natural right to be who you really are. In the Eighth Fundamental T'ai-Chi Exercise, you can feel the prosperous chi energy coming from the earth like a fountain. In the Four Seasons Chi Kung, it may be easy to visualize a tree going through the four seasons of change.

These two exercises are especially powerful if you do them in your own back yard, and better still if you have a small garden. While you are doing the exercise, affirm with your Yin/feminine, Yang/masculine and Tao/creative aspects, 'Infinite prosperity is

flowing to me in infinite ways and I share my prosperity with all around me with wisdom, gratitude and joy! '

The whole universe is echoing this powerful message back to you. You are filled with infinite abundance, talent, vitality, enthusiasm, warmth, clarity, playful creativity and love. You are an enriching being of limitless expression of beauty, precision and joy in every cell in your body right now! Your emotional, physical, mental and spiritual aspects all affirm this inner reality.

Type these words on a piece of paper and stick it in the corner of your mirror. Carry a similar piece of paper in your wallet, too. Every time you read it, it will trigger the powerful connection between your consciousness of the infinite cosmic chi energy that is supporting you and giving you all the life force you need.

I have personally received an abundance of health and prosperity in many, many ways thanks to this affirmation. I know that if you put this idea clearly in your life, it will do the same for you. It becomes a magnet for attracting abundance to you. Have fun. And do share it with as many people as you can. The more you give out, the more it comes around, multiplied a thousand fold!

When you use powerful affirmations in conjunction with the drawing, you are using the universal sound/Yin and universal light/Yang to help you achieve visually what you want in your life.

May chi energy always bring you, your friends and relatives abundant health and prosperity!

The Foundation T'ai-Chi Chi Kung (FTT) course

A long-term training programme for self-development and for becoming an instructor

The Foundation T'ai-Chi and Chi Kung Training Courses described in this chapter build the foundation for deeper work in chi healing. The FTT helps you to accumulate chi energy so that you can channel it into chi healing to help yourself and others. The Trilogue Intensive strengthens your chi understanding and practices with the human condition and spiritual energies.

The background of the FTT, Trilogue and chi healing can be traced to my childhood. As a child, I was intrigued by the art of healing and martial arts. As I have said, my father, Chin Ket Leong, was a Chinese medical practitioner and a martial arts Master. I loved going to his clinic and admired the Chinese herbs in their bottles all lined up on the shelves, with the swords and fighting sticks on the other side. At home, my brothers and sisters and I helped with the drying, grinding, sieving and mixing of the herbs we helped to dig up from the jungle. And when my father saw me developing an active interest in the healing arts, he recommended me to learn with a local T'ai-Chi and Chi Kung teacher, Master Huang.

When I left school and started work, I found myself giving chi healing, chi massage, T'ai-Chi and Chi Kung lessons to my colleagues and bosses. At the same time as I was working, I kept up my study of chi energy.

As a teenager, I also explored the use of the chi force in martial arts. When I went deeper into this area, I became curious about how to apply the principle of self-defence in matters of health. I wanted to learn how to defend myself against my own inner fears, restlessness, nervousness, pain, illness and stress – and help other people to learn it, too. I decided to deepen my studies of chi energy and search for more teachers. I was fortunate to meet wise teachers such as Master Mantak Chia, Professor Jou Tsung Hwa, and Dr T K Shih.

I soon found that whatever I learned from my teachers had some kind of application in my daily life. For example, I felt that there was a correlation between chi meridians and 'ley line energies' of the earth. This made even a simple walk in the city or countryside very interesting. My Chi Kung teachers told me that for thousands of years scholars had claimed that chi is an intelligent energy, and able to express itself through infinite forms. Little did I know those forms included insects.

Those of you who know about chi might like to try this experiment. When the weather gets humid in summer, go into a forest and allow the mosquitoes to come to you. As they zoom in to settle on your skin, just before they start sucking your blood, direct your chi energy the way an acupuncturist would point a needle. Direct the energy to the mosquitoes with peace, then wait and see what happens. If you still feel irritated or nervous or itchy, you need to practise more.

When you can feel your own tingling energy being strongly with that part of your body and the mosquito, I assure you that when your own hair is standing on end (as if electricity were passing through you), the mosquitoes are also experiencing their tiny hairs standing on end! They need to learn to be peaceful, too, and stop irritating me or anyone else.

Another exciting discovery I made for myself is that if you can focus your chi energy on points as tiny as a mosquito bite, you can focus healing energy like laser beams on any part of your body, internally or externally.

I do feel grateful to have found a vocation into which I can put my whole being and enjoy it. I have now been practising these ancient arts of chi healing for twenty-five years and have been training instructors for the last ten years. What is very exciting for me is that my advanced Foundation T'ai-Chi/Chi Kung

Teachers' Trainers Course (F3T) students, Annie Fitzgerald, David Baines, Jeanne Hampshire and Michael Cooke, who are studying chi healing as a vocation to help others, have all produced some beneficial results already. The extraordinary results are based on their understanding of the simple Taoist laws of balancing their Yin/feminine qualities and Yang/masculine qualities first and then extending this creative healing energy to help others.

What is the Foundation T'ai-Chi Chi Kung course?

FTT is a one-year programme whereby participants attend one weekend a month and an intensive summer course in order to achieve a more balanced and healthier approach to their daily lives. Some participants attend it purely for personal self-development, while others work hard to graduate as instructors in the Fifteen Fundamental T'ai-Chi Chi Kung Exercises and Principles. After that there is a year's advanced training focusing on using the T'ai-Chi Chuan classics, the Yang-style T'ai-Chi form and chi healing.

How did this programme start?

After practising and sharing this teaching for about fifteen years, I consulted my teachers and realized that it was time for me to start training instructors. This was about eleven years ago. I had been travelling and studying with seven different groups in Malaysia, India, Scotland, America, France and China. And each centre of learning that I visited developed a certain aspect of myself. I even received an initiation and a new name from each of the centres. So, I wanted to find a path of synthesis. And what better way than to allow T'ai-Chi Chi Kung philosophy and practice to bring it all together?

So, why do it in a group? Because you see the reflections of your being in the other people you work with. As they develop, you too grow. Each person brings his or her humble hope and desire to grow

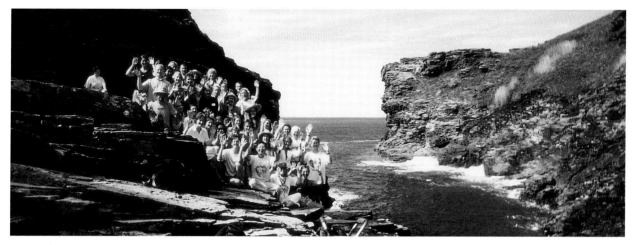

'Power of chi healing' workshop at Tintagel, Cornwall

himself or herself. For me it is literally like watching different trees grow. Each tree is unique and needs its unique environment in which to flourish. This is why, contrary to the fears of some of my students' relatives that I will take them away and create a cult group, we send them back to their families empowered to apply the principles in very ordinary and normal activities. Of course they need to spend time practising the exercises, but this is no different from learning to play the piano or to master the game of soccer. You need to practise, practise and practise. The fruits of your labour are for you, your family and friends to share.

The most important requirement for students applying to join the FTT course is the humility to learn about chi energy. This needs to come from their hearts and must be balanced with a gut feeling that they can trust the chi energy in their own practice and daily life. Students are encouraged to ask questions and find out more about applying what they learn on the course to their daily lives. They must have the motivation to learn to manage their daily pressures and transform their stresses into creative opportunities for personal growth and service to their friends and relatives.

In the Foundation T'ai-Chi/Chi Kung instructors' training, students are aware of this important self-initiative process in their studies. You practise and you get what you deserve. This could refer to the

technical mastery of the exercises or to learning about group dynamics. The instructors themselves are still investigating how they can feel more energy while they are practising the exercises or while they are teaching.

We are constantly challenged as to how to apply the T'ai-Chi Chi Kung principles in an everyday, practical and physical way. New and fresh insights and understanding are always encouraged and written down. Every student has to send in homework detailing his or her emotional, physical, mental and spiritual awakenings.

The most rewarding experiences for me is to see how beautifully and effortlessly the students discover their true selves. It often moves me to tears of gratitude. These true selves are not separate from their daily lives and obligations. But it is when your daily life is at its most demanding that you find out how true you can be to what you believe in. You are like a garden growing the most delicious vegetables and fruits to share with everyone around you. Many FTT students use their new-found knowledge to apply themselves to passing driving tests after failing for ten years; learn to sing or play a music instrument after being convinced for thirty years that they will never be able to; write a book that they have been postponing for ages; or heal an illness which has been disturbing them all their lives!

The articles on the following pages are written by some of my Foundation T'ai-Chi Chi Kung trainees. I wanted to include them in this book to give you a glimpse into how they conduct some of their sessions. Enjoy!

How to understand and apply the Wu-Chi, Yin/Yang, T'ai-Chi, Trilogue and Tao principles in communication

The following is an account of an event that took place between two trainees in an FTT workshop and the instructor. Only the names have been changed.

Mary: But I haven't had much space and time. Everybody else has been speaking and getting attention. I feel I deserve this time to ask about what this Wu-Chi, Yin/Yang, T'ai-Chi, Trilogue and Tao Principles are all about.

Jane: No, no, you have had your chance. Now I want to ask something about this.

Mary (very heated and aggressive): That is not true. I did not, you are wrong . . .

Jane (shouting across the room at Mary): You are the one who is always taking up the group's time . . .

Instructor: Jane, Mary, I wonder if both of you would like to slow down and see what is happening inside you right now. Anne, if you bring your palm up to your heart and the other one to your belly, can you feel the pauses in your heartbeats and your breathing? Mary, could you do the same?

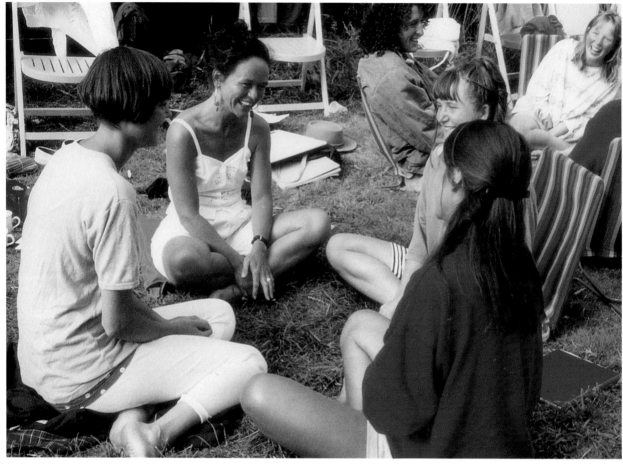

'Tao of happiness and colour science' workshop at Truro, Cornwall

The Yin/Yang swing of one person being very expansive/aggressive and wanting to make the other person contracted/submissive role is an external effort to find the union of Yin and Yang. When you go inside and do it from inside, what happens? When you get angry and upset, the heartbeat listening and listening to the pauses between your breathing immediately help you to get in touch with the universal balancing of Yin-like silences, pauses and spaces between your heartbeats and in-breath/out-breath.

(Jane and Mary calm down.)

Instructor: Now, using the Third Fundamental Exercise and Principle, can you both hold and embrace your inner child and adult inside who are upset. Can you feel that upset part of you, Mary?

Mary: Yes. I don't know how to understand this. I just feel hurt at being ignored and not getting enough attention.

Instructor: Can you just stay with this part of you who is hurt? And can you feel the connection with a pattern that may go back to your parents, perhaps to the way they relate to each other?

Mary: I know my father often squashes my mother emotionally and is very aggressive.

Instructor: This is how we all learn about the way the feminine/Yin and masculine/Yang principles interact and communicate. It is easy to take on the same qualities of Yin and Yang as our parents and behave the same way with ourselves and others. Your Yang/ masculine self squashes and does not listen to

the inner Yin/feminine self, and you find it difficult to be receptive with yourself or others.

Mary: I feel this aggressive part of me taking over.

Instructor: Stay with it. Can you also feel that there is a very weak and frightened part of you there? Hold these two parts with gentleness. Allow them to flow with each other – the powerful and the powerless flowing into a T'ai-Chi dance.

Mary: I know I do this now to my children and my husband. I felt very ignored and lonely when I was a child.

Instructor: Hold that hurt and ignored child the way caring parents would hold their hurt child. Allow the inner mother and inner father to be present. This is the beginning of the Trilogue process of communication between these three aspects.

Jane: Are our inner mother and father our real physical parents?

Instructor: Yes, in the beginning, it is as if your inner family were your original external family. As you work more and more on yourself, you take the best from your original parents and add your own experiences and feelings as you become a parent of your selves. So, there is this communication inside between the motherlike, fatherlike and childlike selves. You can create a more loving, caring and gentle attitude towards yourself and your external family and friends by allowing the change to happen from inside first. The inner mother is nurturing, warm and loving. The inner father represents clarity, patience and the will to serve. The inner child represents joy, gut-feeling/intuition and creative action. Through learning how to slow down and really listen to all these three aspects, you create a more harmonious and peaceful attitude to the outside world. So, if I can come back to Mary. Mary, how are you?

Mary (with one hand on her heart and the other on her belly): I can feel this part of me who has so much pain . . . In the past I have analysed these areas in my life and in some ways I am more tolerant, but I am still easily upset and aggressive with people and I do want to change.

Instructor: Can you take a pause and feel this part who is aggressive? Feel the weak, lonely part too. Feel that inner emptiness, that neediness, the feeling of being abandoned and feeling lost, now. (Pause while Mary does this.) By staying in this emptiness and sinking into it, diving into it, relaxing into it, you no longer need to avoid the void. Every time you feel hurt, you collect little 'holes' and then you get the 'holey spirit'. This 'holey' feeling connects us all to the great vastness of the universe which supports us. During autumn and winter, we see Nature pulling everything into a recycling pattern. One day, one way or another, our entire solar system will be recycled. It could simply be like swirling water in a river pulling every bit of debris and every form of life into it and transforming everything into a greater state of

fluidity. We could just let go and swim with it. The outer swirling black hole has an inner black hole. This inner void is what is called the Wu-Chi. It does not have to be an enemy. By itself it is neither a friend or an enemy. If you dive into it and face it, you can come out of it feeling refreshed and more alive. (Pause.) So, Mary, how do you feel now?

Mary: I feel calmer inside.

Jane: I just want to say to you, Mary, that I am sorry for shouting at you.

Instructor: I don't know if both of you would like to get together and talk with each other more during lunchtime . . .

(After lunch)

Instructor: So, how was it for both of you?

Jane: It's okay. We had a chat. And a nice hug. I was also able to share about it with Tom [another member of the group] and it felt good.

Mary: Yes, I feel good too. I also understand better what Yin, Yang, Wu-Chi, T'ai-Chi and Trilogue are, but what about Tao? What is Tao?

Instructor: When both of you hug your inner family and then you hug each other, you externalize the inner sense of oneness into a sense of completeness. The Tao is this sense of fullness, of wholeness. A small experience of wholeness connects to the sense of greater wholeness.

Application of the Rainbow T'ai-Chi Chi Kung principles conducted by FTT trainees

The following is a transcript of an interview conducted by FTT trainees during their fieldwork training.

FTT Trainee: During a session with three people, I was asked about negative emotions – anger, frustration, etc. They asked me whether it was okay for a Rainbow T'ai-Chi Chi Kung practitioner to a) let her anger out by punching a cushion and b) let her anger out on the person she was angry with! The questioner was concerned that repressing negative feelings, like anger and frustration, was an unhealthy thing to do and she felt it

was better to release any anger she felt directly. She didn't feel responsible for other people's reactions to her angry outbursts. What is the Rainbow T'ai-Chi Chi Kung approach here?

Choy: The Rainbow T'ai-Chi Chi Kung exercises and principles give the angry person another option – you can see and feel that being angry is a role play involving certain beliefs about the person you are angry with. The angry person could punch a cushion or let the anger out on the person she is angry with or she could release her hold on the anger and recall a peaceful self within. This does not mean you are no longer angry. In the Second Fundamental T'ai-Chi Exercise and Principle [see page 30], you have a deeper option, which is to accept the angry self and the peaceful self and try to move towards a more balanced and creative answer to the actual issues involved.

The Rainbow T'ai-Chi instructor can only offer an option – he or she does not have the right to impose the 'correct' attitude on such an angry person. However, if that person decides to slow down and wants to learn the Rainbow T'ai-Chi way to respond to her anger, then we can help her find a more balanced approach using the Second Fundamental T'ai-Chi Exercise and Principle, followed by the Third Fundamental T'ai-Chi Exercise and Principle of learning how to be non-judgmental and forgiving [see page 40]. Then, she may be able to help someone else, like her husband (if he wants to be helped, that is).

Trainee: Should all sessions begin by asking the other person to practise heartbeat listening, even if they are total newcomers to T'ai-Chi, or is it also correct to tune into my heart first and be receptive to their needs, giving them space to chat and feel at ease and then introduce the physical aspects of heart-beat listening?

Choy: If you have the time, yes, do it patiently with the client. Go all the way. If the client wants only an hour session, it is important to balance your timing and include some physical exercises to connect to your client's needs. Take note of the time and of the importance of balancing the amount of sharing and the amount of physical exercising. You can focus on one small piece of information, or on the root beliefs underlying her fear of being let down, starting, for instance, with her pain at being let down in the past. She can learn about self-acceptance and self-forgiveness, in the Third Fundamental T'ai-chi Exercise and Principle.

Trainee: You have said, in relation to the past, that 'you cannot put an end to something that already exists'. You said, 'I am bringing the darkness to the light.' Could you explain this, in relation to the battery process and each person's choice of being responsible for themselves?

Choy: Basically, we all agree (and this includes the scientists) that energy cannot be destroyed. We can break it up, decompose it, transform it and transmute it – whatever, but we can't destroy it. Chi energy is part of everything that has happened to you in the past. You cannot destroy any details of what happened, but a lot of past traumatic experiences can be decomposed into valuable compost for personal development and growth.

For example, how does one deal with depression? In Roni's case, he applied the T'ai-Chi tools and embraced the crying part of him, which was in the darkness of self-hatred, self-punishment, into the light of light-heartedness. Many of you met him and saw how comical he was. He transformed the 'irony' of his situation into a 'Hi! Roni!' attitude. He learnt to be more forgiving, friendlier and gentler with himself.

You cannot destroy the self, because the self is made of chi energy. Your inner battery becomes more energizing when you learn to accept your own negatives and positives and connect it into a creative balance. Just as you need a battery to make your torch shine, you need to make sure your personal batteries are fully charged and ever ready for action. There is a limitless supply of inner batteries within us. We can make our own, so you don't even have to worry about getting them from the local shop!

The search for unity in diversity and the practice of the Four Seasons Chi Kung Exercise and Principle
by Steve Braund, FTT graduate

This session took place at the end of a busy and fragmented day at work for me. I did my best to still myself before making the journey to the house where I had arranged to do the session. I had been told that there might be more than one person interested in taking part.

I arrived to find the family busy, in preparation for a dinner for friends and yes, several people wanted to take part, including one experienced T'ai-Chi teacher from London.

There were a total of four participants: the lady I had made the arrangement with, her fifteen-year-old daughter, her young son and the T'ai-Chi teacher. We looked for a suitable room in which to conduct the session, but found that all the rooms downstairs were too small. We moved upstairs. Aha! A good-sized bedroom. There was another delay as someone went to find a cassette player. Then another delay before we found a candle. Finally the session could begin. No, it couldn't! The youngest son wanted to be in on the action. Why should he be left out?

'You can come in and watch, as long as you are very quiet,' his mother told him. He agreed and the session began. We sat down in a circle, to settle and to listen to our heartbeats. All around us there was a sense of movement and this reflected in the way I was feeling. We could hear the sounds of the cooking downstairs. But we settled into our heartbeat listening. As we began to feel peaceful, the bedroom door burst open. A friend of one of the little boys appeared.

'Hi, can I join in?'

'Yes, of course. Sit down in the circle, next to your friend.'

We tried to continue, to recapture the sense of peace that we had begun to feel.

This was disturbed as the T'ai-Chi teacher had a coughing fit! He had to get up and leave the room, apologizing as he went. By this time, I felt that we had better move on or we would be there all night. My thought was confirmed as the little boy who had just come in found himself feeling too hot and tried to take off his coat without causing any more disruption. The coat seemed to cling to him like a strait-jacket! It made so much rustling and shuffling noise that we all felt unsettled.

At this point, the lady I had arranged the session with started to apologize for the disturbances and chaos. I explained that the situation was a reflection of my own inner state and probably of theirs, too. We stood up and went into the Four Seasons Chi Kung Exercise [see page 100]. They began to focus well, but the littlest boy, sitting watching us on the bed, started to get fidgety and his mother had to leave the room to take him downstairs, to give us some peace.

As they went out, the T'ai-Chi teacher came back in, having recovered from his coughing fit. I then realized that he had missed my explanation of the exercise. I did my best to accommodate him into the group and we moved on.

As soon as we had progressed a little further, the mother came back to join us. By now *she* had missed some of what I had been attempting to explain. Throughout all this activity and stormy energy, I enjoyed an inner smile and felt that it was a colourful reflection of our inner and outer states.

Eventually, we did find some balance between the peace and the chaos . . . accepting both as they were. When the session ended, the children immediately switched to playing their computer games and I was escorted downstairs to meet more of the dinner guests, for a chat and a chance to relax!

I drove home under a huge, all-accepting indigo sky. It said nothing. It said everything.

A session using the First and Second Fundamental T'ai-Chi Exercises and Principles
by Jeanne Hampshire, FIT Graduate and F3T Graduate

I arrived just after Bonnie, my student, had welcomed in a surprise visitor. I hoped that our session would not be delayed. Whenever possible, I arrange my sessions to take place in my own space, at home, so that I can prepare and energize my working environment; but as Bonnie had no transport, I'd agreed to practise this session in her home. I went into the living room and trusted that Bonnie wanted to work with me and would sort things out. Soon after, she introduced me to the visitor, a young man called Paul, and he said he had just become a proud father. He did look very pleased with himself! He cheerily waved goodbye and Bonnie and I settled into our own space.

The session was about 'letting go' and returning to a state of freshness and innocence like a newborn baby.

I've been working with my 'busy-ness'– there's a lot of activity in my life at the moment, sorting out cars and transport, a court case and my daughter Vonnie's birthday arrangements. Bonnie seemed restless and was feeling the pressures of being a mum to a rebellious teenager. I loved and accepted my life pressures and loved and accepted Bonnie and her restlessness.

I felt the First Fundamental T'ai-Chi 'releasing exercise' [see page 26] was the most appropriate exercise to start with, so I excitedly described my new garden compost-bin system to Bonnie and we avidly released all our negativity into it! The negativity was put with carrot peelings, banana skins and slimy egg-shells. My bin loves it all . . . what rich, compostable material. Bonnie's inner teenager sighed rebelliously into the bin!

In the releasing part of the Second Fundamental T'ai-Chi Exercise [see page 30], we started to giggle as we imagined ourselves shaking our arms, hands and wrists close to the ground amongst vegetable peelings and smelly compost! There was a feeling of humour and joy as negativity found its rightful place in the earth.

I noticed the tension lines on Bonnie's forehead visibly soften as we practised the exercise together. The watery, gushing sounds of the tape 'Ocean Dreams' washed over and through us in an atmosphere of serenity and peace.

Bonnie dropped her head and shoulders as she released each arm. I corrected this and put the emphasis on the weight being in the elbow. I supported her arm and allowed her weight to fall to her elbow, before releasing her arm.

Bonnie's legs felt tired and I'd forgotten to mention 'shaking out' her legs. Thank you, Jeannie, for your humility to learn.

Bonnie's arms felt heavy in the first part of the Second Fundamental T'ai-Chi Exercise. This reflected her feeling of heaviness to begin with. She liked the feeling of her hands or palms in front of her face – a lightness. I felt humour, freshness and peace all around us at the end of the session.

A Session with Sally, Kay, Amanda and Penny
by Sue Ash, FIT Graduate

We had the session in a room used for dance and movement. Sally, Kay and I sat waiting for Amanda and Penny, but decided to start without them. We began by focusing on the breath in our belly and a feeling of well-being and of being present and appreciative of ourselves.

When I showed them the first exercise, I could see they were apprehensive. I suggested that they pair up to help each other, to experience the feeling of letting go, as each held the other's elbow and then let go. They found this helpful and seemed to enjoy taking it in turns to be the 'supporter'. However, they were very hesitant about letting any noise out from the belly.

The second exercise was very peaceful for them and they had no hesitation in letting go like rag dolls for the final movement. At this point Amanda and Penny arrived, very bubbly. I accepted them as they were and they settled down quietly. I related the exercises to them. They had come from quite a stressful lunchtime, where one of the residents they were working with kept insisting on taking her clothes off and disrupting things. It was both funny and frustrating for them.

Towards the end of the session, Amanda, who had been inspired by the feeling of new energy, asked if we could end as we had begun, by focusing on the breathing, as she felt it would help her to ground this lovely energy in herself. So this is what we did.

I felt disappointed about the part of the session where we could let go with sounds from our belly centre. The more I focused on the importance of that part, the more self-conscious the others became, so I decided to accept that this was as far as they wanted to go.

The room was fantastic, with a big window giving views of tall trees and fields. I was meeting the part of me who tries to side-step stress and negative feelings with a hyper state of lightness. I was able to be still with the others' energy and encourage them to allow these nervous parts of ourselves to be embraced into the energy. This allowed everyone to relax naturally into a balanced atmosphere.

I really did my best to find my peaceful centre and presentness again, by listening to my heartbeat at intervals throughout the session.

I liked ending the session in the same way as we began. It felt like a gentle finish, because as we focused on our breath, we could hear people coming into the coffee bar outside for a drink and I encouraged the group to extend the feeling of peace to all the sounds outside. It felt like a gentle way to return to the outside world.

A session in the First Chi Kung Exercise and Kidney Chi Kung Exercise
by Jeanne Hampshire

Jenny is in her late twenties and lost her partner two years ago in an accident. She is the vulnerable part of me that has the sense of loss and the part that is inhibited by the past. The session was about healing pain and transformation.

I had got up very early on the morning of the session and looked out of the window. I was given the most incredible gift from the universe – the sky was a velvety indigo, with a full luminous moon shining over the cliffs and sea. The garden was completely bathed in moonlight, the plants and trees casting strong moon shadows. A powerful clarity and stillness emanated from everything. I had the overwhelming feeling that I was releasing the past, yet paradoxically I knew that I was going to remember this experience, that its beauty and power had melted in me forever. I thanked Nature for her gifts and beauty and thanked the precious jewel within myself.

My heart connected immediately to the inner sense of beauty. Jenny shared that she could hardly feel her heart. She had cut off her feelings because of pain and guilt. She was afraid she would not be able to stop crying. My inner child felt the pain and loss of my father and allowed my inner parents to support and love Jenny. My tears flowed with her. I felt my inner child, holding her in my belly with my palms. In the stillness, my inner child felt loved and nurtured. My inner mother and inner father linked hands with my inner child and danced round and round in a circle, 'Ring-a-ring-of-roses'. I shared the image with Jenny and we practised the First Chi Kung Exercise [see page 84] together, pausing to concentrate light in the heart, belly and head.

We both felt a sense of renewal, nurturing and centredness at the end of the session.

A session with Della
by Jeanne Hampshire

An hour before the session Della phoned to say that the friend who was meant to be looking after her little boy, Robert, hadn't arrived yet and couldn't be contacted. It was New Year's Day. Della knew that her friend had been partying the night before and had probably overslept. She was wondering what to do. My kind inner mother self felt like saying that she could bring Robert with her, but my disciplined inner father self felt that Della had the strength to find another solution in order to give herself space for herself.

I suggested that Della could come over half an hour later than arranged, giving her time to sort something out. She arrived, pleased that she had found a willing neighbour to look after Robert. I felt that the quality of strength was the keynote to the session. I appreciated my own courage for being open with Vonnie (my physical child) about having times for myself when I needed to meditate or practise T'ai-Chi. I felt grateful to Vonnie for her understanding and patience.

I felt that this session was 'setting the scene' for a wholesome new year. It felt fresh and full of hope and trust. After practising the First Fundamental T'ai-Chi Exercise [see page 26] and releasing my 'teacher' role play, I was receptive to inner guidance.

Della said that she felt some pain in her lower back, in the kidney area, and that she had 'overdone' eating and drinking over the Christmas period. I invited her to join me to practise the Kidney Chi Kung Exercise [see page 94] and focus on the cleansing aspect of this exercise. The sound of the 'Ocean Dreams' music tape gushed through my kidneys and I released all the poisonous vibrations into the earth. I had recently written about the water contamination incident in our town, so I felt especially thankful for this cleansing exercise.

I shared with Della that this was an excellent exercise for people around this area to practise, because of our water

problems. I was aware that Della had been poisoned. Her kidney pain disappeared and she felt the wonder and joy of the chi energy experience. I felt inspired and humble.

After the session Della and I felt healed, cleansed and stronger than ever in our bodies.

A session in the Four Seasons Chi Kung
by Corazon Wilkinson, FTT Graduate

I was working with a lady called Samantha. I asked her how she was feeling. She said, 'Fine.' Her voice was very shaky. I wondered, 'Are you nervous?' She laughed and admitted that she was. I said, 'Me, too!'

I was holding my heart and belly centres to calm myself and I encouraged Samantha to place one hand on her heart and the other on her belly, to feel her heartbeat and calm her nervousness.

I asked her to tell me a bit about herself. She was forty-six, she lived with her parents, owned a foal and worked in a doctor's surgery. She said she would like to have married and sometimes felt very lonely. She had cancer and needed to have a mastectomy. At this point, she began to cry.

We were silent together. I felt my pain, vulnerability and loss melting with her pain, sadness and devastation. I asked her to be with her pain and her vulnerability.

I first went through the exercise sitting with her. We were both drawing up the supportive, warm, maternal chi energy of the earth and her unconditional love, and we felt our hearts moving through the Four Seasons Chi Kung Exercise [see page 100]. I could see the effort and weight in her hands and wrists, so I suggested she feel that her arm was like a branch swaying in the wind, that her elbow, wrist and hand were one, connected, flowing movement. I asked her to place her hand on mine and follow the lightness. She imagined feeling lighter than air and moved her hand from her elbow. I told her that her elbows were connected to her heart and that her elbows were like birds: that she could release the birds in her heart.

I was very moved by Samanatha's vulnerability and pain. I felt so surrounded by the autumn season that when I went through the exercise, I left the Autumn part out. I felt, 'Oh, shit!' and internally practised the Second Fundamental T'ai-Chi Exercise [see page 30] to bring the opposite parts of me together. We repeated the exercise and I said to her, 'I almost left the Autumn Season out again, I got carried away by the Spring and Summer!'

We both laughed and this created a lovely lightness and openness, as if we were sharing our vulnerability, humanness and humour together.

We paused.

I wondered how Samantha felt about living with her parents. She said that she did not get on well with her father, that he was an alcoholic. I asked if he could sometimes be 'a pain in the neck', and she said, 'Well, yes' in a surprised voice.

I asked about her relationship with her mother. She said they were very different, that her mother did not believe it was important to find happiness. I asked her inner mother how she felt and she said that she felt that happiness was very important.

We paused.

I asked, 'How does the inner woman in you feel about your mastectomy?' She said that she felt sad that she would never have any children. She was crying.

We paused.

I asked, 'Did you feel you repressed any feelings inside you?'

She said nothing, but there were tears in her eyes. We were silent together.

I asked her what her inner child wanted to say about how she was feeling. She said that she was sad and unhappy. We paused, both of us silently being with the sadness.

Then I asked, 'How does your inner child want to be now?'

She said, 'Joyful, happy.'

I said, 'Let's take this into the exercise and feel this joy in your inner child.'

During the practice, I was feeling the wealth of past experiences composting in the earth. I shared this with Samantha. We felt the simplicity of our inner children, as we opened our hearts and our layers of being with the freshness of spring. I could feel my inner smile dancing with the joy of summer. I asked her to let her child's inner smile and joy play and dance. I felt the autumn ripeness and my inner child sharing tears of love, the feeling of my past experiences releasing in the winter and the natural place of death in Nature's life cycle. We felt this, together.

I then asked Samantha to practise the exercise for her inner mother and father and showed her the movement of the triangle and the inner family within the Four Seasons Exercise, so that her inner family could begin to feel the freedom of their natural internal balance, in the cycle of the seasons.

I noticed that her enthusiasm was letting her wrists and hands take over her movements, so I asked her to drop her arm and move only her lower arm from her elbow. I said that her wrists were connected to her mind and that she had firstly to release her mind and move from her heart.

We practised the movement in silence, several times, feeling the natural, flowing movement of the seasons. Then, we paused and sat down again.

I noticed that in lifting her hands from the earth, towards her heart region, they kept connecting together. She found it difficult to keep them apart. I suggested that our body reflects our inner being and that this might connect to her lack of confidence and feeling of vulnerability in her masculine and feminine aspects. I felt that practising this exercise would help her revitalize her natural inner balance

and she might begin to feel the natural strength and individuality of her masculine and feminine aspects.

We practised the exercise, being with the wonderful qualities emerging from our experience together. I encouraged her to appreciate her nurturing support and love, as she gathered energy from the earth: the spring quality of her innocence and openness, the summer quality of her courage and joy, the autumn quality of fluidity in sharing her experiences and the winter quality in her peace and stillness, in allowing herself to release the old for that moment in her life.

I asked what the seasons meant for her and her face lit up as she said, 'The spring is for me a time of new birth, new buds sprouting. Summer is a time for joy and gladness, autumn is for sharing the fruits of summer and leaves turning golden and preparation for the trees to sleep in the winter. Winter is for rest, sleep and death.' I asked her to bring her abundant vision into her experience of the exercise.

Again we practised the exercise several times, in silence, integrating our whole experience for that evening. I thanked her for her sensitivity, her gentleness, her courage to be vulnerable and the whole-hearted gift of simply being.

Becoming a Foundation Taoist and Rainbow T'ai-Chi Chi Kung (FTT) teacher

The teaching programme comes out of more than twenty years of my research into the use of Rainbow T'ai-Chi Chi Kung as an effective, self-empowering and health-directed vocation. It is a one-year course designed to promote self-understanding in participants wishing to share Rainbow T'ai-Chi Chi Kung on a professional basis, as well as in participants wanting to use it to deepen their personal self-development process.

This programme is journey of self-discovery. Anyone from the age of seventeen upwards can apply to join. The only prerequisite is an attitude of receptivity and humility to learn.

The FTT course
The FTT (Foundation Taoist and T'ai-Chi) course is based on the principles of the Fifteen Rainbow T'ai-Chi Chi Kung Exercises and philosophy as described in this book. Unlike other Taoist and T'ai-Chi schools, which focus on mastery of technique but do not fully address the development of the student, this course trains the student to use T'ai-Chi Chi Kung as a mirror for self-development. By mastering the Fifteen Rainbow T'ai-Chi Chi Kung Exercises and Principles, the student first achieves a total sense of personal clarity and acceptance, and then, with skill and sensitivity, extends the wisdom of his or her experience to others.

A journey to discover your true vocation
Many graduates have applied their training to creating happier lifestyles and integrating what they learn into their chosen occupations. The course is also a springboard for many students to discover their true vocations. FTT graduates are much in demand and well known for their holistic, health-oriented approach and the heart, body, mind and spirit emphasis in the way they teach.

At the moment, the one-year intensive course is held at Exeter, Devon, England. The student is required to attend a monthly weekend intensive course and two twenty-day summer intensives. The course normally starts at the beginning of October.

FTT subjects
Course subjects include the Practice, Benefits and Philosophy of the Taoist Rainbow T'ai-Chi Chi Kung Exercises; the Therapeutic Value of Rainbow T'ai-Chi Chi Kung; Leadership Training; Yin/Yang/Tao Balancing Therapies (Thanking Process, Trilogue Process, Option Attitude); CSC (Conserve/Spend/Conserve) Principles; and Small Circulation of Chi Energy.

FTT fieldwork training helps you build up self-esteem, and FTT creative projects are designed to help you succeed in grounding your highest aspirations in your daily life. Students are expected to initiate one-to-one and group participation in weekly classes with qualified Rainbow T'ai-Chi Chi Kung instructors.

If you want to join the FTT course
The first step is to write a letter sharing your intention. The address is given on page 159 of this book. An application form will be sent to you and you will then be interviewed either by telephone or in person. You will be required to attend a minimum of two summer workshops to give yourself a more practical understanding of what the FTT entails. Arrangements for private and extra weekly group sessions are also required, especially for those wanting to graduate as instructors.

The Trilogue Intensive for personal transformation
The Trilogue process is a system for personal transformation based on the use of an inner communication between the Yin/feminine (receptive, mother) principle, the Yang/masculine (emissive, father) principle and the creative Tao (union, child) principle. It emerged from my research into the therapeutic value of

T'ai-Chi, my studies of the Option Healing Process of the Option Institute, Massachusetts, USA, and my understanding of the Thanking Process. In 1986, I blended these three disciplines into the Trilogue Process. Since then, the process has gradually evolved into a valuable art of chi healing and communication.

The training aims to help you discover the true purpose of your life. It will establish a balanced alignment between your personality and your soul consciousness. This linking up of the earth and heavenly energies within you will activate a more creative purpose in your life. It will unblock, clarify and provide a more integrated outlook. You will emerge from the course more confident of your creative abilities and you will find a deeper sense of peace and well-being in yourself and in your relationship to others.

Some of the feedback I have had gives an indication of the effect the training has had on students. Here are just three examples chosen from many:

'The session showed me the concept of the three inner parts – inner mother, inner father and inner child, interacting; actually noticing the imbalance. I was able to pinpoint and follow a feeling back to me again.'

'I found it very moving. I saw that the relationship I had with my inner father mirrored the relationship I had had with my actual father – and I was able to accept both the negative and the positive aspects of that relationship. This felt like a real release and a new awareness, even though it was quite a painful emotional experience.'

'I had a sense of peace and balance between my inner mother, father and child. It was a very heart-centred and joyful session.'

Who will benefit from the Trilogue Intensive?

The Trilogue Intensive is especially designed for candidates who have gone through the FTT and want to use the Trilogue Process on a professional level. This special intensive course will also support their chi healing and F3T work (see below). The Trilogue Intensive is an additional tool for attaining more effective emotional, physical and mental healing when working with clients.

Candidates wanting to use the Trilogue Process purely for their own personal self-development will also benefit from this programme, as the curriculum is centred around the unique requirements of each student; this may connect the Trilogue energy to singing, painting, music, poetry and other forms of performance art. Trainees have used the Trilogue concept to apply and make their artistic ability an expression of excellence and inspiration.

Format of the course

One hour-long, one-to-one session per month is supported by weekly homework of 3-5 hours required of every student. There is also a detailed tutorial in which we examine taped Trilogue sessions and learn how to improve skills in the Art of Listening, Art of Communication, Art of Cognitive Seeing and Feeling, Thanking Process and Option Attitude. Students are expected to initiate their own Trilogue sessions in the practical fieldwork and be able to produce at the end of the training tape recordings of a minimum of ten successful Trilogue sessions.

On successful completion of the course, the candidate is awarded a licence to practice the Trilogue Process professionally in conjunction with his or her T'ai-Chi classes as an extra service to the students. All sessions will be taught on an apprenticeship basis and conducted by me. The training will commence on a one-to-one basis and will run throughout the academic year.

Flexible scheduling

Because of the one-to-one nature of the programme, training is geared towards balancing the work and personal schedules of the candidate with those of the tutor. To enrol, write to me at the address given on page 159, sharing about your intentions in joining this Trilogue Intensive.

Private one-to-one and group sessions are also available

By learning to listen to yourself and to respond in a non-judgmental way, you can create a special atmosphere in which to experience deep calm; this helps you make wise decisions and co-operate with the natural intelligence in your body in any self-healing process. The Trilogue Process complements other alternative health therapies. You will also learn how to open yourself into a more balanced relationship with yourself and experience greater self-respect, care, harmony, support and inspiration in your daily life. You learn how to empower yourself and enrich your life with more creativity, health and happiness.

Besides learning how to listen and calm your emotions and assimilate your past experiences, the session may also include some Rainbow T'ai-Chi Chi Kung exercises and the use of drawing, painting, music and other creative activities. In advanced work, you will also discover energetic dimensions that connect you on many different levels. One of these involves learning how to harmonize the Triple Fire Energy and connecting the Lower Trilogue and the Higher Trilogue Processes. Traditionally in Chinese philosophy, the Triple Fire connotes the chi vital force located in the belly area, the solar plexus area and the chest area. The Lower Trilogue Process involves harmonizing the Yang/ masculine, Yin/feminine and Tao/ creative principles on the human personality level. The Higher Trilogue Process involves circulating the pure Yin/anti-clockwise, pure Yang/clockwise and pure creative energy principles. By harmonizing the Higher and Lower Trilogue Processes, you will be able to attune to more creative energies.

Your Trilogue Process mentor

Each session is attuned to the needs of the individual by a trained and qualified Trilogue Process Mentor who is also a qualified Rainbow T'ai-Chi Chi Kung instructor. Trainees in the Art of Trilogue Mentoring conducting free sessions are usually graduates from the FTT and are personally supervised by me.

Advanced Foundation T'ai-Chi teacher trainer course (F3T)

This is an advanced training programme, designed to teach individuals who have already become certified as an FTT (Foundation Taoist/Rainbow T'ai-Chi Chi Kung) teacher. The programme is held over a period of one year. Upon completing the course and passing the examinations, graduates will assist in conducting FTT courses and will be paid for their professional services.

Syllabus

This is an organic evolving and structured process which includes:

• A thorough understanding of the heart/ body/mind/spirit education system
• Mastering the 37 steps Yang-style T'ai-Chi form and learning how to teach this art of relaxation and rejuvenation
• In-depth study of the T'ai-Chi Chuan classics
• How to use T'ai-Chi Chi Kung partner exercises as a supportive individual/ group dynamic for self-discovery and self-understanding
• Study of appropriate chi energy meridians such as the Triple Burner and heart meridians connected to the Fifteen T'ai-Chi and Chi Kung Exercises and Principles
• Study and practice of the spontaneous chi combustion energies and their connection to the science of effortless chi healing.

The F3T will also conduct on-the-spot training in the art of teaching FTT participants, focusing on the Fifteen Fundamental T'ai-Chi Chi Kung Exercises and the T'ai-Chi Form.

F3T fieldwork

This includes working with a minimum of twenty people in the T'ai-Chi form as well as acting as a mentor to FTT students on a weekly and monthly basis. You will be asked to start a group for the T'ai-Chi form. While giving these classes

Accessories for Rainbow T'ai-Chi Chi Kung

you will emphasize that you are an F3T trainee . To graduate, you need to prduce at least five students who will attend a summer workshop, firstly so that they can demonstrate their mastery of the complete 37 steps Yang-style form and secondly so that you begin to take responsibility for envisaging the dynamics of starting your own T'ai-Chi Workshop Intensives. You will be required to attend two consecutive twenty-day summer courses (see under FTT above).

Additional Direct Chi Healer (DCH) qualification

There will be an opportunity to learn about Group Spontaneous Chi Healing (SCH) and Direct Chi Healing (DCH). To qualify to work as a chi healer, you must by the end of the course show by testimonial that you have successfully healed a hundred students. This qualification is optional. You can still qualify as an F3T graduate and teach the T'ai-Chi form Parts 1-4 without a DCH qualification.

The SCH experience is a natural by-product of a strong chi energy focus in a T'ai-Chi group class, without directly focusing on it as a healing session.

The following accessories may be obtained by writing to the address on page 159.

Laminated footwork charts

To learn T'ai-Chi you need to think along the energy lines from the tan-tien and the limbs. These A3 charts have specially been designed to be used on the floor. They are laminated so that they can withstand wear and tear and at the same time you can see the diagrams clearly.

T'ai-Chi Form Part 1
T'ai-Chi Form Part 2
T'ai-Chi Form Part 3
T'ai-Chi Form Part 4
15 Fundamental T'ai-Chi and Chi Kung (FTC and CK) Exercises with the 12 Primary Chi Meridians
£8.50 plus £1.50 p & p each

Rainbow T'ai-Chi Chi Kung t-shirts and sweat shirts

All sweat shirts and t-shirts are white with multi-coloured design.
Choice of 'Rainbow T'ai-Chi' or 'I Love My Internal Organs' design.
T-shirts £9.50, sweat shirts/pant £25.00 each, plus 10 per cent for p & p (overseas orders 15 per cent). Please state required size (large, medium or small).

Recommended cassette tapes

Exercises
The tapes guide the listener through the exercises step by step and can be used by practitioners who wish to deepen their understanding of the exercises.

15 FTC and CK with Meridians
Tao of T'ai-Chi Story/Part 1 Form
Tao of T'ai-Chi Story/Part 2 Form
Tao of T'ai-Chi Story/Part 3 Form
Tao of T'ai-Chi Story/Part 4 Form
£7.50 plus 50p p & p each

Music
Over the past twenty years, we have searched through thousands of relaxation tapes from all over the world and selected the following. Our criteria are

simple: to find a balance of harmonious sounds (Yang) with pauses (Yin) in between. We also look for a balance between Nature's sounds and human-created mechanical sounds of harmony.

These tapes have been played consistently in T'ai-Chi and Chi Kung classes and have proved very effective in reminding practitioners to relax and return to the gentle, fluid and harmonious nature before starting to do the movements. The rigid environment inside the house or hall begins to melt away and your physical movements flow better. Fluidity is an excellent medium for chi energy. Enjoy the tapes.

'Machu Picchu Impressions' by Rusty Crutcher
A background of environmental sounds which were recorded at Machu Picchu, Peru, during the Harmonic Convergence, August 16 & 17 1987. The music is gently interwoven with melodic textures of Peruvian flutes, drums, synthesizers and natural insect and jungle sounds.

'Ocean Dreams' by Dean Evenson
Dolphins and whales weave their melody with the evocative music of flutes, harps and synthesizer. Gentle ocean rhythms create waves of peace.

'Rhythms of the Sea' by Dan Gibson
A magical blend of piano and surf accompanied by cello, flute, guitar, oboe and English horn, guide you into peaceful coves and along expansive beaches.

'Angels of the Sea' by Dan Gibson
With bamboo flutes, French horn, clarinet, guitar and cellos, experience an under-water concert in conjunction with nine different species of dolphin from the Caribbean to the Pacific.

All the above music tapes are £12.50 plus 50p p & p

'Pace of Peace' by Volker Cat
Soft, ethereal flutes and delicate

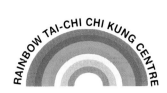

keyboards create misty mountain paths. Ideal music for meditation, T'ai-Chi Chi Kung, massage and relaxation. £8.50 plus 50p p & p

Rainbow T'ai-Chi Chi Kung videos
Thanks to regular feedback from people who have used our videos, we have finally got the ABC Professional Video Makers to make a new version. The viewer will now be able to follow the exercises much more easily because they are shown from back to front, as if you are having a private T'ai-Chi class and doing the exercises along with the instructor. These videos can be used by beginners or advanced students.

8 Fundamental T'ai-Chi Exercises
A concise study of the 8 Fundamental T'ai-Chi Exercises and Principles, shown step by step. The video guides you to learn how to open your chi energy channels. The exercises will help you let go tensions and feel more centred in your heart and tan-tien/belly centres. This is a necessary prerequisite for anyone wishing to study the T'ai-Chi form.

7 Chi Kung Exercises
This video contains information, guidance and techniques about the 7 Chi Kung Exercises and Principles. When followed closely, together with the 8 Fundamental T'ai-Chi video, it has been found indispensable for students attending weekly classes. The video can

deepen your understanding and study of chi energy at your own learning pace. It also includes the Triple Burner Exercise, which has been found very powerful in learning how to channel radiant chi energy to rejuvenate your internal organs.

The exercises on these two videos, taken together, help to build the foundation of an understanding of T'ai-Chi Chi Kung, just as strong and healthy roots support the growth of fruit trees.

Both these videos last an hour and cost £26.50 plus £2.50 each p & p.
Parts 1/2/3/and 4 of the T'ai-Chi Form
Each of these videos continues on from the last. They are recommended for all students interested in using the T'ai-Chi form as a mirror to understand themselves. Part 1 includes the sequence, 'Grasp the sparrow's tail', which focuses on how to harmonize the opposites in your life. Part 2 includes the 'Step back and play with monkey-self' and 'Wave hands in clouds' sequences. Part 3 has an in-depth study of the sequence, 'Golden pheasant stands on one leg', which focuses on learning to channel the energy connecting the earth to the meridian energy along the insides of the body. Part 4 contains the sequences, 'Fair lady weaves at the shuttle' and 'Step forward to greet seven stars'.

All these videos last one hour and cost £36 each plus £2.50 each p & p.

If you have any comments about this book, queries about T'ai-Chi Chi Kung courses or wish to purchase any accessories, please write to

Peter Choy (K C Chin)
Rainbow T'ai-Chi Chi Kung Centre
Creek Farm
Pitley Hill
Woodland
Ashburton
Devon
TQ13 7JY
England

Make sure you include your name, address and telephone number and that the details of your order are clear. Please make cheques payable to K C CHIN. (For orders from outside the United Kingdom, please add 15 per cent to the total amount for postage and packing.) Your letter will normally be answered within 1–2 weeks. Thank you for your patience.

For urgent communications, please telephone Peter Choy 0385 706 965 or 01364 653 618
or by internet to
PETERCHIN1@compuserve.com

Index